Anyone Can Run

Nick Marks

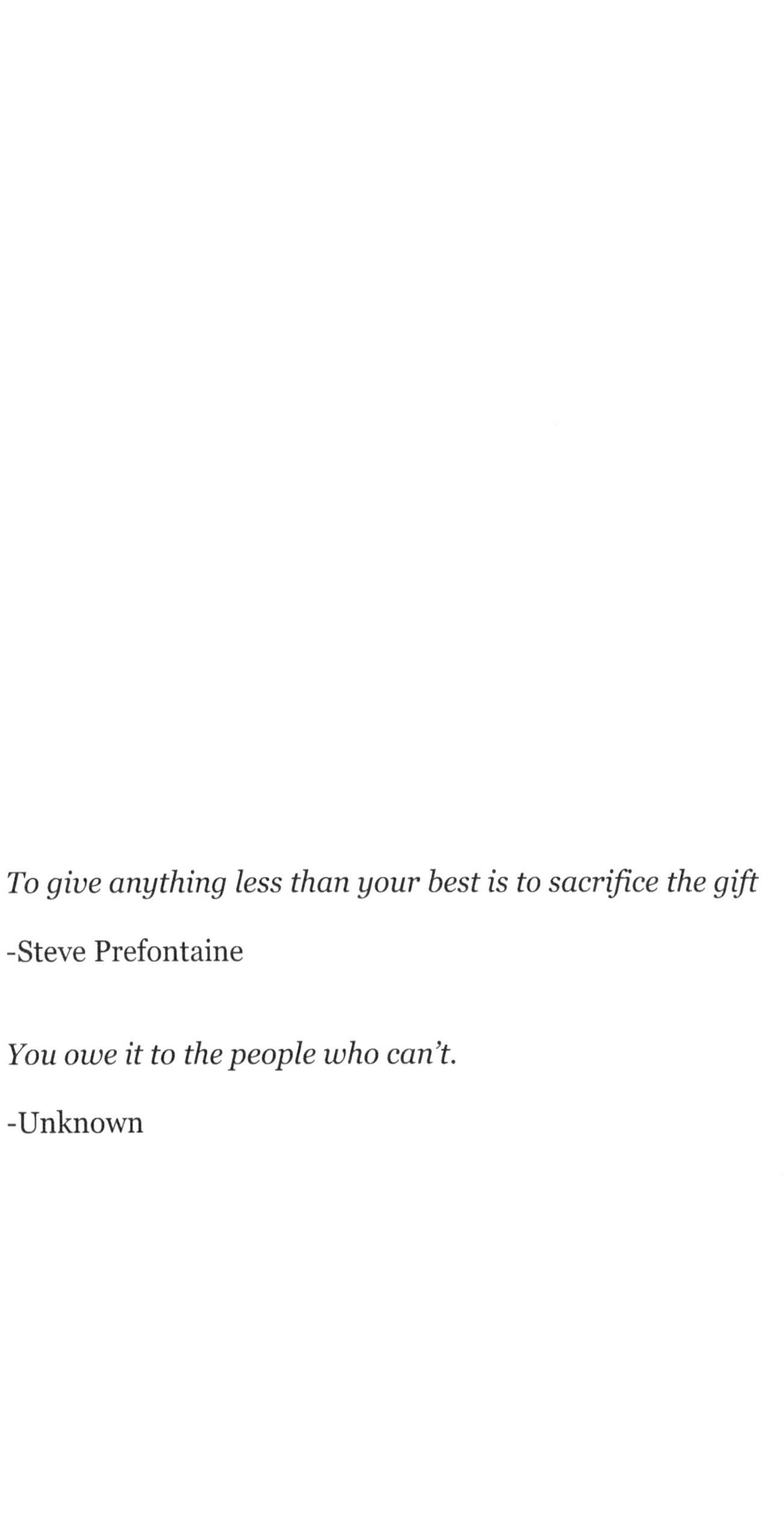

To give anything less than your best is to sacrifice the gift

-Steve Prefontaine

You owe it to the people who can't.

-Unknown

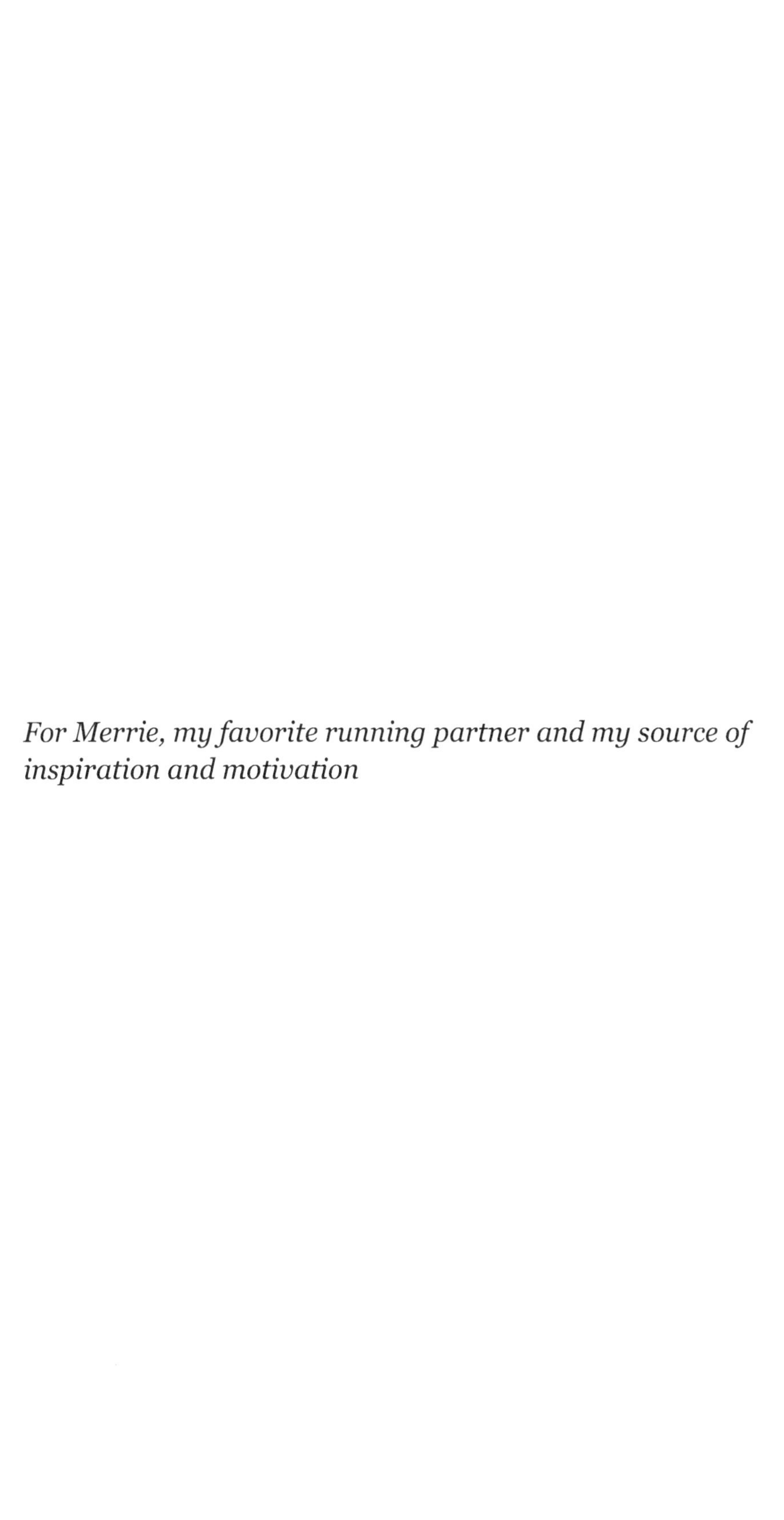

For Merrie, my favorite running partner and my source of inspiration and motivation

Contents

Disclaimer

I'm not a medical professional. Stated another way, I'm a doctor but I'm not *that* kind of doctor. If you're beginning a running plan, or a workout plan of any kind for that matter, be sure you consult your doctor first. This a book for the aspiring runner, no matter what age that aspiring runner might be. But we can't very well have you hurting yourself in your way to becoming a runner, can we? That sort of defeats the purpose.

Introduction

Pain is only temporary.

2016 wasn't a great year for me but I made it my goal to run every day, rain or shine. It wasn't easy many days to add running into an already full schedule, but I made a commitment. I made a conscious decision to try to take charge of at least one aspect of my life. I look back on all those runs that were wedged in between trying to work 10 to 12 hours a day, trying to be a father and a husband, and trying to write a doctoral dissertation. I made it work, but I didn't enjoy running at that time. There are days when it is amazing, and surreal, and magical, and any number of other ways you might try to describe it. On the converse, there are days when you feel like garbage and you just don't want to do it.

That's what this book is about. This book is for the regular runners. The people who have lives, and who decide to run despite being busy. This book is for people who want to be healthy and who want to find a way to run successfully when they've failed before. This book is for people who don't know how to run. This book is for people who want to run better, faster, and longer. In short, this is the book I've been writing for as long as I can remember, through trial and error, success and failure, and constant self-experimentation. It is the book I looked for at the beginning of my running journey that I never found.

This is an 8-week run plan for anyone who is new to running, hasn't run for a while, is coming back from an injury, or needs a templated plan to increase running time or speed. It is a thoroughly tested plan that I've used several times, and it has worked well for me to get me locked into a routine that has allowed me to reach 30 minutes of running every day to build a base. You can decide how it will work for you. There are options for customizability and you can determine your own pace for the plan - how many more runs you want to add during the week in addition to the suggested minimums, what speed you want to run and walk, and what you want to do on the 'in between' days. This plan is NOT a miracle weight loss cure. This plan will not make the pounds fall off. It will make you healthier and set you up for long-term habits that may result in weight loss over time, but the purpose of the plan is to get you out running.

Anyone can run. Many times, we feel like we've missed our opportunity and that because we're not active we need to try other things to either be active or lose weight. And there's nothing wrong with that. But running has its own unique appeal. Running takes you places you wouldn't otherwise go, and down paths you wouldn't normally take. Running can be therapeutic, can help you cope with stress, and can even be a way to deal with addiction. This plan is designed to ease you into running, to build weekly on your run volume in a way that is manageable and to increase at a speed that minimizes risk for injury. Will it be easy? No. Will it take commitment? Yes. But the most important thing about the plan is to stick with it and keep trying. You'll gain confidence as you move from week to week, and before you know it, you'll be accumulating solid mileage. And from there, the sky is the limit. All I'm here to do is to motivate you.

Just get out there and run.

Chapter 0

Getting Ready

Suck it up, buttercup

-Unknown

Are you ready? Are you sure you're ready? Ok. Let's get started.

This will be an 8-week plan, but it requires that you start somewhere. You're starting at 0. Hence the reason for starting the book at Chapter 0. No running necessary yet. You need to be able to walk for 30 minutes. And you shouldn't be straining and pushing yourself to the limit to reach that 30-minute mark.

I'll say that again. You need to be able to walk for 30 minutes at a clip, comfortably. Without keeling over. Because it doesn't get any easier from here.

Other than that, what do we need to do to prepare? There's not much. We discussed a need for a few crucial pieces of equipment - shoes, clothing, and a watch. Each week you'll have a new time goal. This is a time-based plan. We're not worrying about distance and speed. That will come later. For those of you who need to know how much distance you're racking up every week, there's a nifty chart in the appendix that cross-references speed and time to give you the distances for various interval times.

How to Run

Wait a second here. You're telling me that it isn't as easy as putting one foot in front of the other? No, it *is* pretty much that simple. But for you to be successful and to be consistent, there are two rules you'll need to try to abide by. One outdoor rule and one indoor rule. First, the outdoor rule - try to avoid hills and significant changes in elevation while you're on the plan. If you live somewhere that has a topography like the one I have to deal with when I head out my front door, you'll have hills that you'll encounter in nearly any running course you try to plan. I turn left or right out of my driveway and pretty much the first thing I hit is a hill, in either direction. When you're on the plan you're trying to focus on easing yourself in. Hills are a great workout, and they're generally a great means of strength- and speed-building. But they can also very quickly push your body into an anaerobic state. We'll cover the concept of aerobic and anaerobic in later chapters, as well as zone-based heart rate training. For now, I would simply recommend that you try to keep your elevation as consistent as possible to ensure success on the plan. Do you have a local track of some kind? A track at a school, perhaps? A municipal track? Tracks are perfect because you can more easily keep track of your time and distance - they provide a controlled environment with very little change in elevation. Running on a level surface means you're able to consistently focus on your energy consumption. It makes a difference these first few weeks! And while we're talking about tracks, here's a quick snippet of track etiquette. Always run counter-clockwise, and always stay to the outside if you're slower. And try to stay in one lane.

Second rule - the inside running rule. Do you have a
treadmill? Nice. Treadmills can be very useful when it
comes to very specifically regulating speed and time. But if
your treadmill is set at an incline of 0, you're basically
simulating what it is like to run downhill. Here's the rule.
Set your incline at 1. You're trying to give yourself some level
of resistance. It will pay off in the long run. Can you follow
the plan with the treadmill set at 0? Sure. For that matter,
you can negate rule 1 and spend all your time running up and
down hills. Whatever floats your boat. The most important
thing is that you're abiding by the intervals established on a
weekly basis. But following these two rules accomplishes
two things. First, it levels the playing field somewhat
between inside running and outside running. You're
balancing lack of elevation in outdoor running with a bit of
additional elevation indoors to create a consistent level of
resistance between the two. The other thing these rules
accomplish, much more so with rule 2, is that when you start
to run and hit varied terrain, you'll be a little bit more
conditioned to do so.

It can be discouraging, working through 8 weeks of
increasing speed and distance to reach the point where
you're running for 30 minutes at a time, then go outside and
absolutely bonk the first time.

Bonk (verb) - to hit something. As in a wall.

The whole point is to keep things simple and consistent.
Running is putting one foot in front of the other in what is
essentially a controlled forward fall. You're simply picking
up the tempo from your walk speed and exerting yourself a

bit more. If you can control this exertion, you'll be more successful in the long run.

A Few Notes on Running Safety

If you're outside, the number one thing you can and should focus on is situational awareness. Acknowledge what is going on around you. It will keep you from being hit by cars, bitten by dogs, mugged, and from getting in other runners' ways if you're running in a group. I have encountered and/or directly experienced all of the above. I don't obsess about what's going on around me, but I pay attention to noises and motion. I also don't run with headphones on when I run outside. Does that mean you can't run with headphones on? Of course not, but it might be a good idea to run with only one earphone in unless you're in a very controlled environment (like running on a track, which we just talked about). I find that running without earphones not only provides you with a better opportunity to listen to the world around you, but to listen to yourself. You're better able to scrutinize your body and see if anything is out of place, and observe the little tweaks and twinges that might be an indication that you're doing something wrong or you need to dial things back.

I totally get that running with good motivational music can make the run easier and can shift your mindset on days where you're just having a hard time getting motivated to even put on your running shoes, much less get out there and actually run. And don't get me wrong. When I'm on the treadmill, particularly when I'm doing interval work, I love some up-tempo angry music to run to. But when I'm outside I like to enjoy the run. I also happen to live in the woods, so there are lots of obstacles that just sort of show up randomly on the road. Ever run into a moose? I've almost run directly into one, though it happened to be while I was pedaling up a hill on my bike and had my head down. How about a skunk? Yep, nearly stepped on one once. Deer? I've had the ever-living crap scared out of me more than once by a deer crashing through the woods beside me. And I've also learned that squirrels and chipmunks are even louder than deer when they're chasing each other through the leaves. Lots of potential adversaries to deal with.

If you're running outside during the day, wear bright clothing. If you're running at night, wear reflective clothing. These are common sense things, but easy things to forget. The other thing about running outside, if you're running on the road, is WHERE to run. If you're on the trails, that's great. The only concerns you have are wildlife and terrain. Watch out for the death cookies and the baby heads.

Death cookies (noun) - small rocks that you'll encounter on a trail (a.k.a. scree) that will cause you to lose footing and slide around, particularly on uphill (climbs) or downhill (descents) trails. So named because they are cookie-sized.

Baby heads (noun) - these rocks have the same motivation as death cookies, but they are larger rocks that are embedded in the terrain. While death cookies slip around when you run on them, baby heads offer a slick surface that has no give, which means your shoes will hit them and slide off plunging you in unpredictable directions. So named because they are about the size and smoothness of an actual baby's head.

If you're running on the road, you're sharing said road with cars and you need to keep in mind that cars don't always like sharing the road with YOU. Run against the traffic. For those of us here in the US, the cars travel on the right side of the road. Which means you run on the left side of the road, so you can see what oncoming traffic is coming at you. When a car comes, don't expect that the car is going to move over and give you a bunch of room. Be sure to move over to the shoulder as much as possible, but also remember that once you step off the pavement the terrain is less stable and predictable. The last thing you want to do is move to the shoulder to avoid a car, slip, and fall in front of the car. That sort of defeats the purpose of moving out of the way in the first place.

Now that we've got all that out of the way and you're walking for 30 minutes a session (don't lie to me... we'll figure out shortly whether you're telling the truth) let's dig in.

Chapter 1

The Plan

Every day of our lives, we are on the verge of making those slight changes that would make all the difference

-Mignon McLaughlin

Week 1 Overview

Pace	Start Time	End Time
Walk (warm-up)	0:00	5:00
Run	5:00	6:00
Walk	6:00	7:30
Run	7:30	8:30
Walk	8:30	10:00
Run	10:00	11:00
Walk	11:00	12:30
Run	12:30	13:30
Walk	13:30	15:00
Run	15:00	16:00
Walk	16:00	17:30
Run	17:30	18:30
Walk	18:30	20:00
Run	20:00	21:00
Walk	21:00	22:30
Run	22:30	23:30

Walk	23:30	25:00:00
Walk (cool-down)	25:00:00	30:00:00
Intervals:	x8	
Walk	1 minute 30 seconds	
Run	1 minute	
Total run time	8 minutes	
Total walk time	22 minutes	

Assuming Week 0 went well for you, we're ready to move on to week 1. This will be your first foray into specific timed running intervals, for all you newbies. What's an interval? Simple. Something you do for a period of time. We're considering running to be the interval. Generally, when runners talk about intervals, they're talking about the time/speed/distance they're running, and it is assumed that the time between the intervals is occupied by walking or a light jog. For our intents and purposes, there are two speeds involved with these workouts - run and walk.

Give the workout a try and consider how it feels. It isn't going to be comfortable. It won't tickle. It should not be so difficult to complete that you feel you're going to collapse. If you're reaching this point of exertion at any time, STOP. What you're trying to do is sustain activity for a period of time. This first week is crucial in determining what you want your run speed and your walk speed to be. As a guideline, I'll recommend that you choose a speed 2 miles per hour faster than your walk speed for your run speed. If you're starting out and you're a more brisk walker, try walking at 3 miles per hour and running at 5 miles per hour. If walking at 3 miles per hour is too fast for you, try 2. And for that walk speed, you'll be running at a speed of 4 miles per hour.

Make sense so far? Good. Once you're done with your first day's work out for week 1, consider how you feel. You might be a person who journals or has some sort of diary you maintain on a regular basis. Jot down a few thoughts you can refer back to. Here's the point at which you'll decide what format you are going to use to keep track of your running. I'm not asking that you become obsessed over the details, but consider the advantage of having something to look back on if you're having a particularly difficult day and you feel like you're hitting a wall. It is very satisfying to find motivation in the successes of your prior run days.

Don't make any changes after your first run. Give yourself at least 2 or 3 run days before you make a final decision on whether you need to adjust your speed for the rest of the time you're on the plan. Remember, your running needs to be consistent. Your speed needs to be consistent. Deliberate over what you want your final speed to be. You're going to be stuck with it for a little while.

Why We Run

Why do we run? What motivates us? More importantly, how can we justify spending time every day running (often the same paths repeatedly as we become comfortable with them) when we're not really getting anywhere? Do we need to have a reason to run?

We run for any number of different reasons. We run because we want to be healthy. We run because we're trying to find a way to spend time on self-improvement that provides us with an opportunity to de-stress. Some of us run because we find it to be a spiritual or meditative undertaking. Some of us run because it just feels good. It occupies us in ways we might otherwise spend that time indulging in unhealthy behaviors. We run to get away from addiction. To deal with loss.

See where we're going here? You can have any reason you want, or no reason at all, to run. That's the beauty of it. You can be training for a race, keeping up your general health and well-being, improving your fitness without any specific goal in mind. Or you could just be enjoying getting out and getting some fresh air. Pushing your body and achieving the goal of becoming... better. The one universal I think exists for everyone when it comes to running is that it has the potential to make you a better person. What that means for each of us is unique, and that's ok. Running can be different for all of us, and we can come to it for different reasons. You're here and you're running. That's what matters.

Which brings up another question. At what point can someone call themselves a runner? Does it mean you have to 'earn' the title because you've done a specific distance? That you've run for a long enough period without stopping? No. Anyone who runs is a runner. If you've begun the program, congratulations. Let me be the first to bestow upon you the honorable title of RUNNER. Just keep getting up and lacing your shoes, then going out the door and doing it. *That's* what makes you a runner.

Gear

I have a fanatical love of good running gear. Some level of
gear is a necessity, but there's plenty of stuff out there that
just looks too cool to pass up. I've tried a number of different
handhelds, hydration packs, fuel belts, bottles, hats, jackets,
shoes, gaiters, arm warmers, race belts... the list goes on.
And do you know what happens with most of the stuff I've
purchased? It ends up in one of several totes that live in my
garage, because it is specialized gear that I just don't use
often enough to keep it at hand. I've narrowed my gear down
to a few very specific things that are my go-to items, because
my running is consistent, and I've been able to determine
what I need for the volume and type of running I'm engaging
in. It is good to have the additional gear if I decide to change
where or how I'm running, and it is also good to have an
opportunity to try new gear to see if it makes a difference or
suits a particular need for your daily routine. But at the end
of it all, the point at the beginning is to try to keep things
simple. Also, to try to keep the barrier to entry at a
minimum. If you NEED a bunch of gear, that means it is
going to be that much more expensive to get into a regular
routine. Try to get out of the mindset of 'need' and make
sure that the 'nice to haves' aren't ending up on that list.

What You Need and Don't Need

You need running shoes. That's a non-negotiable. Go to a
running store, but also listen to what other runners have to
say. Read shoe reviews. Get on YouTube and check out shoe
reviews. But do so with caution. Anyone can make a
YouTube video, and the vetting of these reviews (and
reviewers) occurs largely out of sight in the comment
sections. But there are some people out there who really

know their stuff. We won't get into the specifics of choosing running shoes (there's a whole section of that coming up) but I will say that you need to be careful in selecting the right shoes.

Figure out what else you need and take a moment after every run to consider the extent to which you actually used the equipment you selected for that run. And did you need it? Or was it extra weight? You don't want to add unneeded weight, especially if you're covering long distances or trying to run at top speeds. If you spend a little bit of time engaging in this reflection, you'll eventually hone your list. I'd still encourage you to try new things, and to give them enough of a chance that you've really arrived at your decision based on adequate time spent with the new equipment. But don't EVER try new things if, down the road, you're running a race. The whole point of these base runs, and of the larger goal of acclimating to running, is to get set in your routine.

Safely Increasing Distance and Speed

The point of this plan is to increase our intervals so you're running more and more each week and walking less and less during a 30-minute session. But what IS a safe increase? The rule of thumb is that increases not be larger than 10% in the course of a week. We're talking about run volume. So let's look at things in terms of round numbers. Say your running for a week adds up to 100 minutes. The next week, you shouldn't be running more than 110 minutes. You're going to encounter times during this plan when the weekly mileage gains might exceed 10%, but since our running volume is fairly low and we're adding running and subtracting walk time, the net amount of time we're spending 'active' remains the same. No worries. Remember, we're just getting used to moving from walking to running for incrementally increasing periods of time. We're not worried about distance or speed.

The Importance of Building Up a Base

What is a base? Well, that's a question that has any number of answers depending on what your goal is. A base is a regularly established amount of distance/time that you're accruing in a given week that provides you with a platform from which you can begin to engage in specialized training focused on either speed, distance, or both. What we're doing over these 8 weeks is creating a base from which we can begin to establish secondary training goals. But we also talked in Week 0 about the need for a base of 30 minutes of continuous walking on a regular basis. Think of it as a series of steps on a staircase. Before you climb to the second step, you need to reach the first step. The fun police won't come track you down if you skip steps, but you'll put yourself at a high risk of injury or failure if you don't pay attention to building up in the right way. We'll talk more about the step approach in later chapters, particularly with the idea of periodization in mind. Big scary words, but not to worry. The concept is very simple. For now, the important thing to remember is that, as with a staircase, you're going somewhere. You're moving up, making progress so you can take the next step. And the next one after that. And then the next one. Just take things a step at a time and don't skip anything, and you'll be ok.

Motivation

Sometimes you have to dig deep. They won't always be good days. You're going to have weather to deal with. Your schedule is going to be full. You'll have other things that take priority, that will push your daily running time allocation to the bottom of the list. How you manage these conflicting priorities is up to you, but if running is important enough to you, you'll find a way to fit it in.

Finding a Reason to Run

Find your reason to run. Figure out what motivates you. Run streaks are a good way to keep yourself on track every day. If you want to make running a regular routine, simply make it a non-negotiable. Every day, have a specific goal in mind. If your goal isn't to run every day, then come up with your weekly schedule and abide by it. But having a schedule alone isn't going to motivate you. You have to find your reason. Does running make you feel good? Does it provide you with an opportunity to indulge in an activity that is selfish, meaning it doesn't have a specific benefit to those around you? Does it make you think clearer? Give you an opportunity to reason through problems? To channel your inner monologue and listen to what your brain has to say to you when you strip away all the distractions around you? You'll find your reason. And that reason will be what keeps you motivated.

Seeking Inspiration from Others

The great thing about running is that we all have so many resources we can tap into for inspiration. It might be friends or family members you know who have had success in running. It might be people you've read about, blogs you've followed, or news stories featuring runners and their accomplishments. There are times you're going to need to be able to tap into others' inspirations to maintain your own motivation, so start now. Running blogs are a great place to start. There are a lot of great ones out there!

What the Pros Say

Books from the pros are a blessing and a curse. We'll talk about the 'curse' part in a second. In terms of the aforementioned inspiration, they can be a great place to start. They take the idea of running and often meet it head-on, while at the same time noting where these people came from and how they became who they are today. I'm a sucker for biographies. I always find them interesting, and the reason for that is because we all started somewhere. We all have some level of greatness in ourselves, and we just have to tap into it. We just have to figure out what parts we need to work on in order to achieve our goals. And we all need to realize that talent might be lurking inside ALL of us. Talent isn't just born. It doesn't just happen. It is cultivated.

The Problem with Emulating the Pros

So now for the 'curse' side of the coin.

There are so many different plans out there. So many different people who have the 'best' approach to how to do something. Is the plan in this book the best plan out there? Heck no. I'm sure there are plenty of others that are better. Is it a well-tested approach? I'd like to think so. I've seen a lot of success in this plan, both in myself and in others. I've also come across plenty of plans that sound great in theory but fall apart in practice. The most difficult advice to put into practice can be the advice that comes from the people who are best at running. The pros. There is so much knowledge to be had, so much wisdom to be gleaned from those elite runners who make a living running any number of distances at any number of speeds. The problem isn't them. The problem is us.

An elite runner is dealing with a plethora of data while he or she is running. Fatigue is being monitored in so many different capacities, hydration, exertion, and the elusive 'drive' to keep going. We all have drive. But this drive manifests in all of us in different ways. I guarantee you, Ryan Hall is not thinking the same thing I am when I run. He's not considering the same variables. And that's perfectly fine. Meb Keflezighi, the same. And it isn't because he's in another league. He has invested a lot of time and effort to become who he is from the standpoint of sheer physical ability, and that's not to say that we couldn't necessarily rise to a similar stature. But we're all at different points in the journey. There's no magical training plan that we can all universally pick up that will provide us with the knowledge and skill necessary to run a 2:10 marathon. That comes from somewhere else.

Is it bad to read these books, to review these plans, and to incorporate this wisdom into our own running? Of course not! Devour these plans, read these books, and follow the wisdom of these elite runners. But know that you're not going to find a magic bullet. There's not one universal approach because everyone arrives at their level of achieved skill by different means. Realize that the inherent danger is in measuring yourself against the abilities of others. You're running your own race, and ultimately you have only one competitor in that race. Yourself.

Discipline

Discipline and motivation are two different things. Motivation is having the desire to do something. Discipline is doing it consistently over time. I'm *motivated* to do a heck of a lot, but my self-discipline is another thing altogether. Sometimes we have grandiose plans of where we want to go and what we want to do, but in the end, we need to create a system of discipline to actually get those things done.

The great thing about running, though, is that with more running comes more of a desire (motivation) to run. And if you maintain discipline, then you're going to advance. If you're motivated but undisciplined, you're not going to advance. This plan takes discipline, and you'll get out of it what you put into it.

Self-Coaching

One other thing to consider, as we work our way through Week 1. Self-coaching is an option for some, but for others it just doesn't work. Running groups can help to create accountability, but they can be a difficult thing to be involved in as well because everyone is on a different page. Rarely, in an all-comers group, is everyone matched up. You'll feel frustrated if you're always the one in the back of the group. If you're the one in the front of the group, everyone will be annoyed that you're always running away from everyone and not slowing down in order to keep the group together. When you've got the right group, it can make a huge difference.

We're talking about initial running training, though. So it
has to be a partnership or small group that is specifically
focused on that goal. If you need an accountability partner
to make this work, that's completely ok. Try to figure out
what you need in order to make things work. But
understand that if you slack off, the only person you're
disappointing is yourself. I wish I could be there to coach
you, I honestly do. I know you can do it. I have faith in you.
But you have to have faith in yourself as well, and to know
that at the end of the day you're going to have goals you're
going to have to hit if you're going to want to advance to the
next week. It's right around the corner. I can see it from
here. Are you ready?

Chapter 2

Routines and Making Habits

You either ran today or you didn't

-Unknown

Week 2 Overview

Pace	Start Time	End Time
Walk (warm-up)	0:00	5:00
Run	5:00	7:00
Walk	7:00	8:00
Run	8:00	10:00
Walk	10:00	11:00
Run	11:00	13:00
Walk	13:00	14:00
Run	14:00	16:00
Walk	16:00	17:00
Run	17:00	19:00
Walk	19:00	20:00
Run	20:00	22:00
Walk	22:00	23:00
Run	23:00	25:00:00
Walk (cool-down)	25:00:00	30:00:00
Intervals:	x7	

Walk	1 minute
Run	2 minutes
Total run time	14 minutes
Total walk time	16 minutes

Forming Routines

How's it going so far? What do you like or not like? I'm not just talking about the running plan. It hurts, and it is going to hurt. When we as runners reach that fabled runner's high, there's nothing to match it. But you've got to put in a bit more time before you get there. Let's focus on the now. How do you feel? Is running creating an opportunity for stress relief and self-indulgence, or is it stressing you out? If it IS stressing you out, why? Is it the plan itself, or fitting it in?

The structure of the plan is such that the beginning of each week is going to be the hardest. Then the subsequent runs for the remainder of that week are going to feel easier. You'll ramp up the next week and it will be tough all over again. Remember the step approach we were talking about? Bingo. That's it. But every week you're putting the same amount of overall time aside for your weekly sessions. If you're stressing, I'm going to bet it might be because you're having a hard time fitting it in. You're making a change, and you need to adjust your schedule to accommodate that change. I get it. Let me see if I can help. After all, it's what I'm here for.

Time Management

We're all busy. We all have things we need to accomplish in the course of a day and we're all up against trying to do it all in the same 24 hours we're all allocated. Here's a magical thing you'll find out over time - running will give you more time. I can hear you naysayers out there right now - *But Nick... I'm having to sacrifice things in my schedule in order to run. So how am I saving myself any time?* You're making yourself healthier. You're running, and the more you run regularly the better you're going to feel for the majority of those hours in between running when you have other things to do. One of the best ways to increase productivity is to take care of yourself. Prioritize your running so you can fit it in every day, and you'll reap the benefits long-term.

Look at the things you're trying to do during the day and figure out where you have some 'give' in your schedule. I'm going to be unpopular with the next thing I say, but it must be said: you probably spend a LOT of time on social media. No? Not me, you say? We're all guilty of it. I have met very few people in my life that don't carry a phone and find themselves using that phone as a go-to when they need to occupy a few idle minutes. That programming gets in your head over time and you begin to accumulate things you like to do online. Those things end up becoming part of your regular routine. Check Facebook. Check your Twitter feed. Hit up Instagram. I get it. That stuff is a great way of remaining connected, and I'd go so far as to say it can even help you stay motivated if you're a runner (there are TONS of very extroverted runners out there who are very accomplished and very proficient – some even do this running thing for a living). You simply need to stay within the boundaries you have available. Manage your time based on your obligations and consider running to be one of those obligations. Work, family, running, eating, sleeping. Those are the sorts of things you need to consider prioritizing. We'll talk about non-negotiables in a minute, but I want to be sure we're on the same page from a time management standpoint. It is totally possible to fit it in. I run, I write, I'm a dad, a husband, a teacher, a college administrator, and a homeowner constantly having to fix things around the house. I find a way to fit things in. I have a very rigid schedule and I abide very strictly by the time management rules I've set for myself and I make it work. But it isn't enough to just tell you that you need to be better about managing your time, is it? Would it help if I gave you some organization tidbits as well? Ok, baby birds, I'll feed you.

Organization

If you're going to be organized, you need an organizer. No kidding, right? Thank you, Captain Obvious.

Don't worry. I'm going to give you more than that. What I mean is that everyone has to have an organizer of some sort in the meta sense - a WAY of staying organized. Here's what I do to stay organized, so feel free to take whatever you want to for ideas on how you can build your own system. I have two calendars I use - a work calendar, and a non-work calendar. For my system, my tracking of things is fairly binary. I have work items, and non-work items. And the two DON'T MIX. I have figured out over the years that compartmentalization is very important. We don't all have that luxury, but whenever possible you need to work while you're at work, and don't work when you're not at work. Look at your 24 hours and pull out the time you'll need for work and commuting. You'll use that time according to your work calendar. For your non-work calendar, you need to establish a time you'll go to sleep and a time you'll wake up. Pencil these in, because they might change according to what you need to accomplish during the day.

Try to define a period in which you'll accomplish your running, and try to make it the same time every day. There are four times it will be, for most of our schedules. First thing in the morning, at lunch, after work, or before bed. The earlier you can do it in the day, the better. The end of your day should be about relaxing and winding down. Running ramps up your system and then you might find you're having a tougher time falling asleep. Or maybe for you it actually has the opposite effect, and it helps you to relax and makes you feel tired. Wonderful. Figure that time out for yourself and go with it. I won't judge.

For the non-work stuff, my wife and I keep a shared Google calendar. We have two active school-age boys and we need to be able to have a system for remembering what happens on what nights, what school activities are coming up, when the field trips are, when to make lunch... all that stuff. Since most of that stuff occurs during regular waking hours, I just get up before anyone else and get my stuff done first thing. I fit the running in as close to the beginning of the day as possible, so I don't have it weighing on my mind all day. Because then I'll just start to dread it, and I'll be frustrated when I finally do get a chance to run after working all day and I'll feel like garbage the whole time.

Use whatever system works for you. The calendar will be for events, then you'll use a task list prioritized by immediate, short-term, and long-term designations. This list will be prioritized by 'need-to-be-dones,' and 'it-would-be-nice-if-there-were-time' items. Also known as negotiable and non-negotiables.

The Importance of Non-Negotiables

Non-negotiables can be a good thing. They can keep you on track. Too many non-negotiables can create stress in your day though, so be mindful of the number of non-negotiables you have. If running is one of them (and it should be, if you're trying to follow any sort of plan) you might need to jettison one of the non-negotiables. This can be tough, but take a step back and look at your daily routine for a moment or two. You might have phantom non-negotiables on the docket every day that you're not aware of. Let's consider that routine you have in the evening of putting your feet up and relaxing while watching a television program or two. If you do that every night, there's something right there you can avoid. Here's a proposed solution for you. Don't watch the program(s) at night. Instead, record them, and go to bed earlier than you normally would. Then get up, earlier than you normally would, and you can watch them WHILE you're running (assuming you're running on a treadmill). See there? You're multitasking, you're getting your running out of the way early in the day, and you're not missing out on your programs.

I'm not one who likes idle time. It makes me feel guilty, like I should be doing something. As a result, there's very little time I have that I would find to be dedicated to doing nothing. But I do have plenty of things that waste my time and leave me struggling to address my non-negotiable list during the course of the day. That's why it is important to start with the 'need-to-do' list before those time-wasters

swoop in and ruin the day for me. If I can't get things done
and I have to wait until the end of the day to address my
daily list, then I'm totally stressed out and none of it ends up
being quality time.

How to Make a Habit

So how do we make habits? Repetition, but not just that.
Focused repetition. Trying to recreate the
event/task/objective as closely as possible every day. That
means the same time (hopefully), the same preparation, the
same execution. Doing things in this manner for a two to
three-week period helps to ingrain habits. Breaking a habit
is a science in and of itself, which is why our to-do lists
usually don't get smaller but rather continue to increase in
size. But making habits can be a relatively simple process. If
you mess up and miss a day, it isn't the end of the world. But
always consider WHY you missed a day, if you were
supposed to have a particular thing to do. We always have
things come up that make it difficult to reach our goals. But
if we're missing them regularly, then we need to consider
whether we're taking the right actions to form the habit.
Same time, same conditions, over a period of time. Practice
makes perfect.

Eating the Frog

This is a technique I've used for a number of years now with
varying levels of success. I'm a procrastinator at heart, so I
will often avoid important deadlines because my monkey
mind is intrigued by other things. Sometimes it seems like
*any*thing can often be more inviting than the task at hand. It
is one thing to say you're going to sit down and write, and
entirely another to become distracted with something else.

Writing, for me, is a very spontaneous thing. I have ideas and I need to be able to capture them at any time because that's just how my mind works. I'll chug along and find I'm thinking in the back of my mind about something, and it interrupts my train of thought for whatever it is I need to do. So how do we deal with managing these intruding priorities? We eat the frog. We take the most difficult, daunting, nasty tasks on the list and get them out of the way first. We do this so they are not compromised later when we're trying to add them on top of whatever else has transpired during the day and taken us in whatever direction we're going to go.

Consider a boat, anchored in the water. Wind and currents influence where this boat is going to go, if it isn't anchored. When we get up in the morning, we pull up the anchor. We're going to go where our environment takes us. Therefore, we need to make the most of the time we're anchored and try to get things done before we start getting pushed around. We 'eat the frog' and take a bite out of the nastiest tasks we are going to have to deal with during the day. And for me, I make running a frog. I don't consider it a nasty thing to have to deal with, but I also don't want to be pushed around later in the day, so I get it out of the way. I have days where running truly is a nasty undertaking and something I don't enjoy, but I do it anyway. I eat the frog.

Planning Your Day

If you can lay out your day so your frogs come as close to the beginning of the day as possible, all the better. This doesn't always happen. Also, I don't know about you, but my weekdays are very different from my weekends in terms of obligations. I always have plans to keep things as consistent and organized as possible on the weekends, but inevitably they are nowhere near as organized as my weekdays.

Why is that?

The busier we are, the more we have at stake so the more organized we have to be. And the more organized we are, the better we're able to lay out our day so that everything lands where we want it to. Lay out your day in such a way that your goals will be achievable, and they'll be enjoyable as well. Running should be something you enjoy (more on this in a minute) so why not give it the time it deserves? Put your morning together in such a way that you're able to get up and get everything done without having to rush around. Have a cup of coffee and wake up before you run, but don't go hopping onto your phone or tablet. Compartmentalize your morning so you have the luxury of controlling what you're doing. Here's a suggested schedule for the day in a nice and easy to follow bullet format, based on how I approach a workday:

- Get up early
- Make a cup of coffee and don't get on any screens
- Journal for a few minutes, and if you find things are already starting to come to mind that you'll need to add to your to-do list for the day, create a parking lot for them and revisit them later
- Change into your running clothes and make sure you have everything you need for the day's workout
- Go run
- Journal your run, if that's something you do
- Grab a shower
- Get ready for work
- Drive to work

- Work
- TAKE A LUNCH BREAK
- HYDRATE WHILE YOU'RE AT WORK
- Come home and leave work at work
- Eat a healthy dinner and spend time with your family
- Destress, and try to make the night relaxing and recreational

Now, is there one single day in recent memory that follows that plan? Nope. I'm afraid not. More likely, I'm shuffling things around and using my evenings to try to get everything done. But there are a few things I do as consistently as I possibly can, and running first thing in the morning is one of them.

Prioritizing Running - Investing in Yourself

Don't consider running a drudgery. If you do, and you find this is your overwhelming opinion of running, perhaps you should try other forms of exercise. Running, when it becomes a regular part of your life, isn't a routine. It is time for yourself, where you invest in an enjoyable endeavor and just have a bit of your day to yourself. It is an investment that pays dividends, but those dividends aren't always apparent. It can take time to fall in love with running. If you do, when you do, you'll know it. Because you'll find there are other times during the day when you think to yourself, *I'd rather be running.* Or you're thinking back to the morning's run. Or already looking forward to the next run. And when this happens, you're no longer having to struggle to prioritize your running. Quite the opposite, you're having to consider what things on your to-do list will need to go so that they don't get in the way of your running!

Life Happens

I've said it before. Life happens. You deal with it and you move on. If you're missing a day here or a day there, it is normal. It is going to happen. If it is only a day, simply repeat the training you were going to do that day, the next day. Say I'm on the second week of the running plan and I have a presentation I have to leave early for at work, so I miss my morning run. Then I have to work late, or there's something else going on that night, and I can't run that night. The next day, I'll do that run I was going to do but that I missed. I'm technically a day behind, but I'm not really losing ground. Losing ground is something that happens when you miss a chunk of time over multiple days. You can't always pick back up where you left off, depending on the amount of time you haven't run. There's no magic number on how many days you can miss before you start to degrade in performance and will need to move back to prior weeks' plans. I'd say if you're missing huge chunks of time it points to a larger commitment issue you might need to address. But I'd say over a week, as a guideline, would be a very bad thing in terms of inhibiting progress. If that happens, I'd recommend rewinding one entire week.

Sleep

I've mentioned it before, but we all end up having the same 24 hours we need to be able to work with in a given day. What percentage of that needs to be sleep is something that is highly varied from individual to individual. Some of us need 8 hours of sleep. Some need 10. Others might do ok with 5 or 6. But the important thing is to keep in mind that this block of time needs to be preserved. Look at it as a block you could potentially move around. Not a block you could subdivide, though there are a number of studies out there on polyphasic sleep and the idea that you can break your day's sleep into smaller chunks across a 24-hour period. For simplicity's sake we're going to talk about one solid block you can move around a few hours back and forth in order to accommodate your schedule.

My recommendation is to go to bed earlier and try to get up earlier. You'll find you have more time to yourself because, statistically, everyone else isn't getting up as early as you and when they ARE getting up that early, they're doing so for the same reasons you are. They're taking time for themselves. They're carving a piece of time out of their day that they can use for focused work before they have to start doing all that other work that needs to be done during the day. If you want to realign your day in this way but you're deeply entrenched in a schedule involving a late bedtime, it is an easy process. Set your alarm five minutes earlier. Take a few days to become acclimated to that newer waking time, but also remember that it means you're setting your bedtime for five minutes earlier. And try to your best to stick to that. After a few days, move it another five minutes. Come up with a specific approach that works for you and, as with your running and many other things in your life, try to be consistent. Give yourself a five-minute adjustment every five days, for instance, and see how you do with that.

I can't stress this enough. Sleep is one of the most important things you can provide for your body, and I can attest to the fact that as a long-suffering insomniac I've had many issues with health and wellness that have improved with the more time and effort I've spent on sleep hygiene. And no, sleep hygiene doesn't mean taking a shower before bed or sleeping with clean sheets. Indulge me one more simple bulleted list before we move on to the next chapter.

- No screen time for the last hour before you go to bed. The last two hours...even better.
- No alcohol for the last two hours before bed. We'll talk more about this when we talk about diet.
- No heavy exercise for an hour before bed.
- Find something to do that will relax you. Read a book, but make it something that is easy to digest and won't get your brain pumping and thumping. Nonfiction is good.
- Go to bed when you feel tired. And if you go to bed and you don't feel tired, get up for a little bit.
- Don't go to bed and read or play on your phone. Go to bed and sleep.
- Set your phone some place out of reach, so that you can't easily snag it at night and wake yourself up, and also so you will need to get out of bed to shut off the alarm.
- Sleep in a dark, cool, quiet room.

That's pretty much it. There are tons of other pre-bedtime rituals you might try that will improve your sleep and there are others that are just a waste of time. If a warm glass of milk (yuck) is your thing, or a mug of chamomile tea, go for it. But unplug and destress first and foremost.

Chapter 3

Diet

Success is the ability to go from one failure to another with no loss of enthusiasm

Winston Churchill

Week 3 Overview

Pace	Start Time	End Time
Walk (warm-up)	0	5:00
Run	5:00	8:00
Walk	8:00	9:00
Run	9:00	12:00
Walk	12:00	13:00
Run	13:00	16:00
Walk	16:00	17:00
Run	17:00	20:00
Walk	20:00	21:00
Run	21:00	24:00:00
Walk	24:00:00	25:00:00
Run	25:00:00	28:00:00
Walk (cool down)	28:00:00	30:00:00
Intervals:	x6	
Walk	1 minute	

Run	3 minutes
Total run time	18 minutes
Total walk time	12 minutes

How are you feeling this week? Feeling like you're kicking butt or dragging butt? Either way, you've made progress and you're here! Let's move onward and upward and talk about ways to make sure you're fueling yourself right so you can get everything you can out of your runs.

How to Eat Right

Oh, the rabbit holes we could go down when we talk about diet. So many options to choose from, so much to avoid. So much time wasted calculating how much of this and fretting over getting not enough of that. I'm going to keep it easy for you, and hopefully demystify the process for you so you can actually start worrying about other more important things, like whether those yellow running shoes are 'too' yellow, and whether you can get away with wearing more than one fluorescent color at a time (spoiler alert - of COURSE you can wear more than one fluorescent color at a time!).

Here's the big secret. Are you ready? Is there anyone looking over your shoulder? Can I tell you this in confidence? After all, you and I have spent three weeks together, and I feel like we're really starting to connect. This is special information, just for you. Here it goes.

If you're following a diet, you're doing it wrong.

Wait, what? But you just said I'm supposed to eat right?
How can I eat right if I'm not on a diet? Simple. If you're on
a diet, it indicates that you're pursuing that select group of
foods, cooking methods, and eating habits for a *period of
time*. You're going to 'diet' as a means of reaching a
particular destination. But proper eating is the JOURNEY,
not the destination. We're talking about eating right
permanently. Get the idea out of your head that there's a
special diet out there that is going to magically solve all of
your problems. Because while it might work in the short-
term, the only way it will truly work is if it works long-term.
And that's not a diet. That's called a lifestyle.

Tricked you. Sort of. What I'm trying to say is that you need
to get beyond the idea that you can only have this or that.
Unless you're under a specific dietary restriction, the idea of
restriction is going to work against you. You do not have
permission to eat whatever you want, whenever you want it.
Let me say that again. Step away from the Twinkie.

What I'm suggesting is a set of rules by which you'll govern
what you are allowing yourself to have most of the time and
allowing yourself to indulge once in a while. Do you want to
have a candy bar? Ok. But you realize that if you have a
candy bar every day, you're adding to your daily caloric
intake and your body is only going to burn a certain amount
of the calories you take in during that day, right? The rest of
them get stored as fat. And we don't like fat. Fat is not cool.
Fat makes us feel... fat. Lethargic. Unhealthy. And it puts
us at risk in SO many ways. Cardiovascular health is just one
of the main risks. Consider the impact your added weight, if
you weigh 50 pounds more than someone who is your exact
height and approximate build has if you're pounding on your
feet and legs while you're doing interval runs. Connective

tissue is at risk of being compromised. As in, you're going to
hurt yourself, so knock it off.

The rules are simple. What's more, there are plenty of non-
diet diets out there. Lifestyle changes, if you will. Rules by
which you'll decide on a daily basis what is and isn't feasible.
Go to the references section and look at a few of the books
I've included in the food section (not the *diet* section - we're
not going to say that word anymore) and allow me to draw
your attention to two excellent books that outline the concept
of rules pertaining to eating. The first is *The Skinny Rules* by
Bob Harper (2012), and the second is *The Four-Hour Body*
by Tim Ferriss (2010). I'm telling you to check these out not
because they provide the specific information you need but
rather because the context of these two books is rules.
Simple guidelines that are easy to follow can help you on
your way to making a lifestyle change. Not a diet change.

When it comes to these rules, we're not talking about things
that are way outside of the box and are revolutionary new
ideas. There aren't many original ideas here because, let's
face it, we've pretty much reached full saturation on ideas
out there when it comes to eating. It is the tried and true
that make the cut and end up being en vogue, because they
never really go away.

Balancing Nutrition

Start by looking at what you're eating. For everything you
pick up and get ready to put into your mouth, question how
much processing has been undertaken to put that food into
the form it is currently in. The less processing, the better.
Too much processing, and what you're left with isn't really
even considered food anymore in some instances. Start with

identifying if it is food. If it passes the initial test, make sure it occupies one of the following categories - vegetables and fruits, healthy fats, and protein. We're not going to dispute the merits of eating vegan over eating meat, or over eating keto instead of high-protein. Or Paleo or any of that other crap right now. What we're talking about is simply balance. Fill your plate up with vegetables as much as you can and eat lean proteins and healthy fats. Keep it simple. Stay away from carbs that are just adding calories. "But I'm a runner, and runners need carbs, right?" Runners that are running particular distances need particular types of carbs at specific times. We're keeping things simple.

Hydrating

It can be hard to reach consensus on the amount of water we're supposed to be drinking on a daily basis. Let's just arrive at an amount and you can feel free to adjust it up or down according to your needs. 64 ounces. 8 glasses of water, 8 ounces per glass. That's a nice round number. We're talking about plain water or sparking water without artificial sweeteners. Artificial sweeteners are chemicals that generally aren't good for you. Avoid them. There's also some science in there that we won't go into, focusing on the fact that taking in artificial sweeteners still prompts insulin production in your body. Plain water, as much as possible. Not diet soda, or a bunch of sweetened juice, or anything else that is going to have anything more than what you need. The more you drink plain water, the more you're going to find you actually like it. Particularly after a long hot run.

What to Stay Away From

Stay away from processed grains and pastas specifically. There are tons of pasta options out there that have varying levels of good/passable ingredients, but generally you're going to still be taking in some level of ingredients and additives you don't need. Want some spaghetti? Try spaghetti squash. Excellent substitute. Find the reason you like pasta, and then try to find vegetable substitutes that still scratch that itch. Make changes a little bit at a time if you need to but try to avoid empty carbs. Also try to avoid dairy. Dairy has protein, but the payoff isn't worth it when you look at the calories associated with milk and cheese. You need to be careful.

Remember as well that when you go down a path and make decisions not to eat particular things, you're going to want those things more than ever because they suddenly become forbidden fruit. And when you have an opportunity to eat some of the bad things, you want to eat ALL the bad things, because they're a gateway to old habits that die hard. The word you want to become familiar with is 'moderation.' Moderation is the difference between a tablespoon of peanut butter and a ladle-full. Moderation is the difference between a bit of milk added as an ingredient when you're cooking, or just chugging a pint of milk on its own. Try to moderate a bit.

Alcohol and Caffeine

Uppers and downers. Ouch. These can create a vicious cycle that is difficult to impossible to get out of unless you completely break your routine. We're busy people and we have a lot to do, so it isn't uncommon for us as functional human beings to bring ourselves 'up' to the demands of the day through gratuitous applications of caffeinated beverages. Choose your poison, we all have some sort of drink we drink to start the day. Those of us who do not have caffeine as an ingredient in said drink are the fortunate few. For the rest of us, there's nothing that can beat the energy of a good cup of coffee or tea, or an energy drink.

Yep. I'm right there with you.

Here's the problem, and it is a very simple problem really. You drink caffeine to get up. You spend all day being productive and trying to cram as much in as possible, then you get to the end of the day. And it can be hard to come down. So what do many of us do? Have a glass of wine or two, or a few beers or mixed drinks. This is the vicious cycle. Uppers to get up in the morning, and downers to get down. Alcohol is a depressant, but it doesn't just relax you. There's a lot going on that you don't consider. Alcohol dehydrates you. It is empty calories, so you're just drinking calories that have no nutritional value. It messes with your metabolism, which in turn can have a negative impact on your sleep. It can also make you do stupid things, in large enough quantities.

Is it bad to drink in moderation? If you're a person that is wired up to be able to do so, enjoy that glass of wine here or there. Sparingly. But if you're like me, one or two glasses isn't usually enough. That's why 0 is the right amount for me. I still drink caffeine in the morning, but I'm also conscious of the specific amount I take in and I have a threshold I don't allow myself to exceed. This is in overall dosage as well as timing. No caffeine after noon for me. Find what works for you. If it is a case of not being able to sleep at night, consider how much caffeine you're taking in, and/or whether you're also drinking alcohol at night. Give yourself an hour before bed for each drink you have. One drink? You should be done with it an hour before bed. Two drinks? Two hours. This provides a good starting point for you. More than two drinks? Naughty, naughty. Try to avoid more than two drinks, and definitely avoid two drinks every night. Weekends? Perhaps. I'm not giving you license here to spend a lot of time and effort trying to come up with an elaborate program of what you are allowing yourself to drink. I'm simply calling your attention to substances that you need to be careful with. They can inhibit your productivity and make it difficult to get up in the morning to do what you want to do.

Drinking Your Calories

Here's a simple one. Unless your drinks are protein drinks or vegetable drinks (and one can argue the actual and perceived health benefits of vegetable-based drinks), stay away from drinking your calories. You should be eating real food as much as possible, so supplementing is generally only something you'll be doing if you're trying to SUPPLEMENT the food you're taking in. This means either you're missing out on a time you'd otherwise be eating, and you have to go with some healthy substitute, or you're not getting a specific nutrient in the food you're eating. Consider your diet before you consider adding caloric drinks to your regimen. And for the love of all that is holy, stay away from fruit juice. It has vitamins, I know. But it also has a LOT of sugar. And sugar is something you're trying to cut back on.

Diet drinks, you say? No. I'm afraid not. Chemicals, you see. Far too many chemicals and processing. Just stick to water, either still or sparkling, and natural flavors. There's a product out there called Real Lemon you can get, and you can add it to water for a bit of flavoring. That's all you need at this point. In the future, we'll be talking about electrolytes and the dangers of depletion over long periods of running, but that's not you yet if you're on a beginner plan. Half an hour isn't enough time to deplete your body of electrolytes. You'll be ok. Take a knee and drink water.

Thoughts about Carbs

We're bringing it all home now, food-wise. We've talked about a few basic rules that will provide you with parameters from which you'll begin to craft your own specific dietary preferences. You know what to examine if you're not moving in the right direction on the scale, keeping in mind of course that this isn't a weight loss plan. This is a running plan.

What about carbs, then? Are they really that bad? When it comes down to it, no. They're not. They're not as evil as we make them out to be, but that's because most of us have no control when it comes to carbs. The actual amounts of carbs we can reasonably allow ourselves to eat, based on basal metabolic rate (the amount of calories our bodies burn when we're sitting around doing nothing) combined with exercise is a *very* small amount of the larger picture of the plate we should be consuming. Think about your dinner plate, ala the FDA's recommended daily allowance of food categories, and remember that your plate is going to be vegetables and protein, with fats sparingly. And sugars sparingly. Grains are taking the place of other, better calories you could be eating. More nutrient-dense foods. Don't try to convince yourself that just because your pasta is colored green or vegetable-based, it is going to be a satisfactory substitute.

Instead, look for ways you can substitute vegetables for pastas, like we've already talked about. Your body will thank you.

When to Eat

Finally, let's talk for a moment about scheduling your meals. There are varying opinions on the best schedule to follow when eating, and they all oppose one another significantly. Is breakfast the most important meal of the day? Is it better to skip breakfast? One large meal at the end of the day? Four smaller meals evenly spaced across the day? I wish there were one right answer for this, though the best approach is to spread your meals out throughout the day to ensure you're taking in consistent calories and not creating caloric spikes during the day. You need to find what works for your schedule, but more importantly you need to find an eating schedule that allows you to moderate. You should not be so hungry, when you reach your established meal time, that you're going to eat everything in sight. Most of us have issues with portion control as it is, and when we're even just a little hungry that goes out the window. Smaller meals, evenly spaced calorie intake, and moderation. That's the key. If you want to tweak from there, I'd recommend looking at the concept of intermittent fasting. I've used this approach in the past with varying levels of success.

Chapter 4

Vitamins and Supplements

Nana korobi ya oki (fall down seven times, get up eight)

Japanese Proverb

Week 4 Overview

Pace	*Start Time*	*End Time*
Walk	0	2:00
Run	2:00	7:00
Walk	7:00	9:00
Run	9:00	14:00
Walk	14:00	16:00
Run	16:00	21:00
Walk	21:00	23:00
Run	23:00	28:00:00
Walk	28:00:00	30:00:00
Intervals:	x4	
Walk	2 minutes	
Run	5 minutes	
Total run time	20 minutes	
Total walk time	10 minutes	

We're making progress. You're up to 20 minutes of running this week, so this is the point during the plan when things start to feel difficult. Remember, the pain is temporary. That's the feeling you get when weakness leaves your body. Let's build on last chapter's discussion of food and focus more on how you can effectively build up your body to be in optimal running health.

Multivitamins

To take or not to take. That is the question. And a loaded question it is. There are so many supplements out there, and so many vitamins to choose from. What do you do? Here's what you do to keep things simple. In fact, we already talked about it when we talked about diet. Try to get as much nutrient dense food as possible during the day that will have these vitamins in it already. If you're adding vitamins, it is because you're not able to eat food that provides said vitamins. The exception is vitamin B6, which is not a plant-based available option. For those of you out there who are vegan, you'll need to take this supplement. For those of you who are meat eaters, you're good to go.

That leaves us to sort through the ominous shelves of supplements that we see whenever we walk into the vitamin / minerals / supplement section of the local grocery store, mega-store, or nutrition/vitamin shop. We can debate the merits of some of these substances, many of which are not necessarily FDA-approved and definitely not FDA-endorsed. Generally, the fewer pills you can get away with taking on a daily basis, the better. Try to avoid fat burners, diet pills, energy pills, and things of that nature. Often these things might have some short-term gains, but they'll wreck long term havoc on your cardiovascular system and could also create nerve damage. It depends on what substances, what studies, what side effects, and who is marketing them in which markets. The world of supplements is a huge place, and a very lucrative industry. Try to avoid supplements. Keep it simple. Real food.

What Supplements to Take and What to Avoid

So now that I've said that, there may be some supplements worth taking that you might want to look into. Not because they are miracle drugs, but because they do have some properties that might help you along without creating long-term issues.   Melatonin, perhaps, for those of you who don't sleep well at night. St John's Wort for balanced mood (though this is unconfirmed). Cumin, for anti-inflammatory properties. Be intelligent about the supplements you decide to take and do your research. If it seems too good to be true, it likely is. After all, if it does what it says it does, why doesn't everyone else just take it for the miracle cure it actually is? Stackers were a supplement that, for a long time, seemed to be a miracle cure for energy and optimizing workouts. However, they did so at a price. I don't think anyone wants to sacrifice the various systems in their body in the interest of a little bulk or a little less fat, when you can do the same through just investing some time in taking care of yourself. If you use your energy to engage in things like running instead of seeking drugs as a shortcut, you're going to live longer and be healthier. You have to work at it.

This also goes for things like creatine and weight-gain/muscle-gain products. Your point is to engage in aerobic activity. Aerobic activity does not inherently 'bulk' you up. It provides an opportunity to burn fat and to tone muscle. Try to get your protein from natural sources, but certainly take protein supplements if you're not getting enough protein. Don't take protein for purposes of building muscle though (and by building muscle I mean bodybuilding).

Thoughts on Cleanses and Detoxifying

Tread lightly in the land of detox and cleanses. Many of these cleanses involve significant caloric deprivation. While it can be good that you're avoiding foods that have been contributing negatively to your health and well-being, avoiding all foods and engaging in a juice or special soup cleanse can be dangerous. Talk to your health care professional about ways you can safely detoxify. Cleanses and fasting can be a good thing, but do your homework. I'm not endorsing any of them, or telling you that you should go out and do a cleanse. In fact, I'm telling you not to.

Instead, consider what you're eating and what you're putting into your body on a daily basis, and whether those substances are truly healthy or unhealthy for you. There's a fairly binary approach to this - either they are, or they aren't. The one exception is things you think are healthy but that you are either adverse or allergic to. In those instances, if you can engage in a food allergy study to determine whether you have any specific aversions to particular foods or chemicals that occur within foods, it is a great idea to get tested. We can experience inflammation and health-related issues from eating foods we don't know we have sensitivities or allergies to, so if we can identify what these foods are and avoid them, we'll be much better off!

Pre-Workout Supplements

I'm of the opinion that, for this plan, you don't need preworkout supplements. You don't need a bunch of energy going into a run because you're going to drive up your heart rate and that's going to impact your aerobic threshold. Don't worry, there is a whole chapter on heart rate training coming right up. For now, just understand that when you take supplements that are designed to give you 'more energy' they are stimulants and might impact your ability to regulate your exertion over the course of a run. You're much more susceptible to going out hard and then bonking or redlining right away in terms of your heart rate. You're actually going to find that this makes the run harder for you, and you're not going to have a quality experience. Do you wake up with a cup of coffee in the morning? Fine. Do you happen to have that cup of coffee before you log your morning run? Also fine. But do you have the cup of coffee in order to give you enough energy to be able to run? Not fine. If you don't have enough energy, you need to look at other things. Are you getting enough sleep? Are you eating the right foods? Are you hydrated? Making sure you hydrate is going to provide a very positive payoff, particularly first thing in the morning when you get up. My suggestion is to avoid preworkout supplements. You just don't need them.

Chapter 5

Heart Rate Training

Live like a clock

Bruce Denton, Again to Carthage

Week 5 Overview

Pace	Start Time	End Time
Walk	0	2:00
Run	2:00	10:00
Walk	10:00	12:00
Run	12:00	20:00
Walk	20:00	22:00
Run	22:00	30:00:00
Walk	30:00:00	32:00:00
Intervals:	x3	
Walk	2 minutes	
Run	8 minutes	
Total run time	24 minutes	
Total walk time	8 minutes	

How are you feeling this week? At this point you are making great progress and should be starting to feel like the runs are starting to get easier. If they're not, why is that? Well, let's look at some of the concepts of heart rate training and see if we can figure it out. We're going to keep this chapter short and sweet.

The 80/20 Rule and Training at Lower Paces and Distances

Running is generally NOT a great way to lose weight, unless you're going about it the right way. Sure, your increased activity is going to increase your metabolism and you're going to see your body getting leaner if you're fueling yourself with the right food, but I don't recommend running as a weight loss plan. What I do recommend is running as a means of building cardiovascular fitness. The loss of weight is secondary. The point of this chapter is to give you an edge on fat loss, on running more efficiently, and to give you some pointers on how you can begin to develop the skill of listening to your body and knowing when to increase or decrease intensity in your running regimen. And it starts with a heart rate monitor. If you don't have one, GET ONE. This is important, because the data you get from your heart rate monitor will be essential to dialing in your training as well as troubleshooting where you're going wrong.

With that said, let's rub some science on this and see if we can make sense of all of it. First, let's look at the concept of max heart rate. Have you ever seen this equation before?

220 - age = target (max) heart rate

This is an equation that has been used to establish, based on age, that you can calculate your max heart rate based on strenuous cardiovascular activity. So, if I'm 40 years old...

220 - 40 = 180

The problem is in what we do with this math. Does this mean that 180 is the number we need to try to hit if we're training? Some references to this equation call the number a max, and some call it a target. What's the right number?

There are two types of running. There's aerobic running, in which you're sustaining your run over a long period of time at a lower heart rate. There's also anaerobic running, where you're basically running all-out for a short period of time and you're running at a deficit of oxygen. You're running at a point where your body can't bring in the amount of oxygen it needs to sustain your run. Think sprinting.

Of these two, we're trying to focus on aerobic running. We want to have enough gas in the tank to be able to finish whatever distance or time we're setting out to run. In order to do that, we need to keep an eye on the data to figure out if we're pushing the needle over the line and edging into the anaerobic zone. There's nothing wrong with this for interval training, but we're not there yet. We'll cover that idea in Chapter 9. For now, we want to keep our heart rate low enough that we'll be able to sustain our run by burning fat.

But wait, you say. Burning fat? I thought you just said that running was a bad way to try to lose weight? Well, I stand by what I said. You shouldn't take up a running program simply because you want to lose weight. But you CAN lose weight as a positive side effect in a safe manner if you make a little modification to the equation:

(220 - age) x 0.8 = target heart rate for aerobic activity

So, if I'm 40...

220 - age is 180. I take 80% of 180 and I get 144. That is the number I need to worry about (your number will likely be different) when I'm running. That is the point at which, if I go over it, my body will no longer be burning fat and will instead be burning glycogen. We store glycogen in our muscles, and there's a finite amount of it that we can burn off at a given time. Once it is gone, we're done. No more activity to be had utilizing that form of energy. If we keep the heart rate lower, it allows our body to instead tap into fat stores. I've included a chart in the appendix of this book to make it a bit easier for you to identify your own target and max heart rate numbers. Just look up your age, and you'll see your corresponding numbers.

Why is all of this important to us? Let's end with that. This is important because you're going to feel sometimes like running is hard, and sometimes feel like it is easy. You're going to want to push yourself, and you're also going to have days when you won't be able to bring yourself to run. If you're watching your heart rate data, this can be an indication of when you need to adjust your running speed and distance goals. As a general rule, if your average heart rate at the end of a regular/aerobic run is well above your target, you are likely running too fast or for too long a period of time. If it is well below the target number, you could stand to reasonably increase your speed or time.

There are other factors that influence heart rate besides distance and speed. Elevation is another one. Do you live in a hilly area? Try running on flats, or around a track, and see what the difference is between your average heart rates for the runs. You'll find it is significant. Do you feel like you redline when you race? It might be adrenaline from participating in the race and getting caught up in everyone else's pacing. Run the same course if you can at some time other than race day and see if your average heart rate changes. Observe your heart rate, but also have fun running. Heart rate data is information you can use to your advantage, but there's a lot to be said for just going out and enjoying your run.

Breathing

One other thing we need to keep in mind as we're running is that it is an aerobic activity - we're breathing while we're doing it, and we're trying to sustain the activity by taking in oxygen. But the amazing thing about our running ability as human beings is that we can vary our breathing. We can breathe quicker or slower, depending on the intensity of the run and how much oxygen our bodies need. And the quicker we breathe, the quicker we burn energy, if the mix isn't right.

If we're running and we're trying to keep our heart rate in that target zone, we shouldn't be gasping for breath. We should be breathing comfortably enough to sustain the activity. As soon as we start to breathe too quickly, our body begins to shift into anaerobic mode. In order to breathe the right way, we need to pay attention to cadence. Cadence, simply put, is how often your feet hit the ground while you're running. Left foot, right foot, left foot, right foot. 1, 2, 3, 4. When you're running, count when your feet hit the ground. If you do this for a minute, you'll arrive at your cadence per minute. If we're trying to run aerobically, we shouldn't be breathing in and out every time our left or right foot hits the ground. Instead, we should be breathing at a pace where we're breathing in and counting off 1, 2, 3, 4, and then breathing out for a count of 4. Left foot, right foot, left foot, right foot... that should be an intake of breath. Then left foot, right foot, left foot, right foot... those next steps should be an exhale of breath. Try that and see if it helps. Or stretch it out even further. If what we just described was a 4-count, see how your breathing works out if you do it for a 6-count. Experiment to find what works for you but know that the steadier you breathe, the more you're naturally decreasing your body's tendency to run at a higher heart rate for a given activity.

Chapter 6

Positive Visualization

Never judge your life by one bad day. Judge your life by the best day.

Sebastian Kienle, Ironman World Champion

Week 6 Overview

Pace	Start Time	End Time
Walk	0	2:00
Run	2:00	14:00
Walk	14:00	15:00
Run	15:00	27:00:00
Walk	27:00:00	30:00:00
Intervals:	x2	
Walk	1 minute	
Run	12 minutes	
Total run time	24 minutes	
Total walk time	6 minutes	

Good Times, Bad Times

Running is an amazing phenomenon. There are days when you're running when you'll feel like you're on top of the world. You'll have unlimited energy and feel like you can run forever. You'll be truly unstoppable. Then there are days when you'll have to drag yourself out of bed, throw on your running shoes and slog through painful miles. Your feet will feel like they weigh a ton, you'll be sluggish, and it will take everything you have in order to get through your miles for the day.

Why is this? How can it be that we feel great one day, and terrible the next? We talked about this in the last chapter, in terms of ways we can keep an eye on data to make informed decisions about whether we should step things up or slow things down. But the terrible truth is, we just have good days and bad days. Running is like anything else in life - inconsistent at best. We do what we can to keep our training as consistent as possible in order to minimize these bad days, but they still happen. The important thing is to not get discouraged. Things get better. Just keep at it, and you'll see.

Hitting the Wall

You WILL hit a wall. At some point when you're running, you'll find that you reach a point when you can't keep going. It happens to everyone. When it happens, it can be quite inopportune. Maybe you're having the race of your life, hitting a pace you've never hit before, and suddenly you find that you're just out of gas. There's nothing left in the tank. The trick is to use these opportunities to examine what you're doing and figure out the reason behind hitting the wall. The way we learn is through making mistakes and reflecting on them. Does hitting the wall mean we've made a mistake? No, not necessarily. But it does present us with a great opportunity for reflection. What were we doing in the days and weeks that led up to that point? What did we do while we were running that was different? What external conditions (heat, wind, precipitation) might have been different? Did we have the right gear for these external conditions? The trick when you hit the wall is to ask questions. Sometimes it just happens, but oftentimes there's a reason (or two, or more) behind it that gives us an opportunity to improve what we're doing so we don't do it the next time.

Being Consistent

The trick to all of this is to just be consistent as much as possible. Try for the same time every day. Try to prepare yourself in the same way. Use the same equipment. Fuel and hydrate yourself consistently. What you're trying to do, in being consistent, is to remove as many variables as possible from the equation so you can better identify whether there are things that are different on a day to day basis that might be impacting your running.

Don't underestimate the impact of stress on your running routine. If you're dealing with stress in your job, your personal life, or anything else you're trying to deal with that might leave you feeling like you're unable to deal with it effectively, chances are it will manifest itself in some physical way. We're animals. If we encounter stress, our bodies react. The amazing thing about running is the healing power it can have when we're trying to deal with stress. Running can be an opportunity to unplug from things, to set them aside for a little while and just focus on ourselves. Commune with nature. Give our minds a chance to just *chill out.*

Battling Through and Breaking Through to the Next Level

It takes perseverance to get through the bad times, but it might also take a change to your routine. If you're finding that running is more difficult and you're trying to be as consistent as possible, begin to change the things you're doing consistently. It could very well be that those things are contributing to the problem, not the solution. For example, if you're consistently running in the evenings, try running in the morning. Having a hard time breathing while you're running? Pay attention to your cadence and try to adjust your breathing to see if it helps. Having a hard time running around your house? Consider the elevation you might be encountering and seek flatter terrain for a little while.

Don't give up. You'll get there. Sometimes you have to regress, to slow things down or dial distance and time back, in order to make gains. We'll talk about this concept more in Chapter 9 when we discuss periodization. Bottom line - you'll have plateaus or 'walls' you'll hit as you continue your journey. How you overcome them will largely be through persistence. Decrease your speed and distance if you feel you need to, but don't stop. Take your established rest days but don't add to them (unless you're injured). It is easy to begin to add more and more rest days, and before you know it your butt is planted firmly on your couch while you munch on potato chips and bemoan the condition you're in, longing for those bygone days when you were once a runner. Do you want to be a runner? Then keep being a runner. Just keep doing it, and you'll find that those insurmountable obstacles end up being something you can only see in your rearview mirror as you continue to make forward progress.

What Works for Some Doesn't Work for Everyone

Years ago, my wife was running regularly and was experiencing a number of issues with muscle soreness, joint fatigue, and overall inability to make any progress with increasing distance or speed in a sustainable way. She went to her primary care physician to seek treatment, and for an explanation of what might be going on. The response she received?

"Running isn't for everyone."

How much more discouraging can you be to a person? That stands out for me as the single most obtuse and ignorant response I've ever heard from a licensed medical professional. Are there people out there, who due to specific irreversible medical conditions, are unable to run? Yes. My wife was not one such person, though. I stand by the message I'm trying to convey in this book - everyone can run. The difference is in how fast, how far, and how long. If you can walk, I present the argument that you can run. The motion itself is not so different. What counts as a run for one person might be nothing more than a shuffle to another. But if we look at the definition of running in a broader sense - motion that you're engaging in that is faster than the pace at which you walk - it gives us a starting point. From this, we can begin to improve our locomotion and make progress in the land of running. We can be fit individuals, and we can enjoy running for the many benefits it provides us beyond simple aerobic fitness. Mind, body, and spirit - running can

truly be life changing if we can get beyond the caveman
mentality that running isn't for everyone!

The Fun Afflictions Runners Experience

We runners face unique afflictions that can leave us sidelined
if we don't address them. Shin splints, plantar fasciitis,
iliotibial band issues, back pain, knee problems, chafing...
the list goes on and on. We're talking in this chapter about
being positive and battling through those times when you
feel like the runs are hard. But sometimes they are hard
because of injuries. STOP RUNNING IF YOU ARE HURT. I
can't overstate the importance of this. Don't be macho and
try to finish a race if your knee tweaks. If you roll your ankle
while you're out on a training run, don't keep running.
Positive visualization is something we need to embrace in
those times when we need to dig deep and find more than
what we think we might have. It is not an opportunity to
further damage your body if you experience an injury.
Statistically, if you're a runner, you WILL hurt yourself at
one point or another. It might be a repetitive motion injury.
It could be an accident. It could be any number of random
things that leave you sidelined. I always abide by the RICE
approach when dealing with an injury:

Rest
Ice
Compression
Elevation

I also seek medical attention as quickly as possible to ensure
that any of these measures (ice specifically... sometimes it
can do more harm than good) are not making things worse.
If there is a requisite amount of time you need to take off

from running, take it. You'll be up again before you know it. But if you start back too soon, you'll pay for it in the long run.

Clothes Fitting

I've said in previous chapters that running to lose weight is a bad thing. Run first, and be consistent, and you'll see the weight come off over time. Your clothes will begin to fit more loosely, and this can be a huge boost to your confidence. Positive motivation isn't just in how we're feeling at the time we're doing something, and a means by which we can try to get through the tough times. We can also positively visualize over time based on the improvements we're able to observe in ourselves. Weight and inches lost can be great motivators. It can be hard to see these things on a daily basis, and indeed I discourage the general practice of weighing yourself every day because you'll see too much up and down motion on the numbers of the scale to be able to observe trend data. I would instead encourage you to take your weight one day per week. You'll see better results and a more encouraging trend this way, if you're doing things right. And I have a feeling you *are* doing things right, if you're doing your best to be consistent!

Reaching Your Goals

What are your long-term goals? Now that you've been running for a number of weeks, start to consider what comes up next. Want to run a 5K? A 10K? A half-marathon? The sky is the limit. You'll continue to make progress. In the meantime, keep an old pair of pants around to try on once in a while. It can be very encouraging to put on that old pair of pants and see how much more room the 'old' you occupied in

them. Remember, this is the NEW you. You're a runner
now. And the nice thing about being a runner is that it
doesn't take a particular distance or speed or amount of time
you run daily to be considered a runner. We're a very
welcoming tribe, and we like to see our own out there doing
it. Period. Keep doing it, and even if you're not fast or able
to run for very long... you're still a runner.

Chapter 7

Strength Training

-You should actually limber up as well, especially if you're going down that hill. It's very important.
-I don't believe in it. You ever seen a lion limber up before taking down a gazelle?

Columbus and Tallahassee, Zombieland

Week 7 Overview

Pace	Start Time	End Time
Walk	0	2:00
Run	2:00	17:00
Walk	17:00	18:00
Run	18:00	33:00:00
Intervals:	x2	
Walk	1 minute	
Run	15	
Total run time	30 minutes	
Total walk time	3 minutes	

The Importance of Strength Training

As runners we often forget or underplay the importance of strength training. We run, so we strengthen the muscles we need to use while we run, right? Wrong. In order to more effectively run and to keep ourselves injury-free, strength training is an essential thing we need to practice regularly. As you run, you actually create imbalances in your muscles based on the motion of running. You're pushing/pulling consistently with some muscles, but not with others. The more you run and the stronger you become, the more you risk injuring yourself. What's more, running in and of itself is a high-impact activity that can damage your body if you don't balance it out regularly with other activities.

At this point in your training, begin to consider other exercises you can incorporate to prevent these injuries from occurring. We'll discuss a number of options in this chapter. These are easy exercises that in some cases might only take a few minutes a day but will pay you back immensely in ensuring that you're able to run efficiently and safely. There are things you can do that don't take specialized equipment, so you don't have the excuse of not being able to get to the gym!

Cross-Training

Running is an impact-based activity. There's no way around it. Whether you're running on the road, running on softer surfaces such as rubberized oval tracks, or even if you're using a treadmill with shock absorption build into the deck, you're pounding your legs and giving your body a fair amount of abuse. Part of minimizing this abuse can be addressed through running technique, and we'll cover this briefly in the concepts of specialized equipment as well as in Chapter 8 when we discuss barefoot running. But part of it can also be minimized by substituting cross-training opportunities for some of your run days.

If you're running every day, consider taking every other day and engaging in a different activity. These substitute activities can offer as-good or better calorie burning options, elevated heart rate, and sustained cardiovascular opportunities. Elliptical machines are a great low/no impact way to go. Cycling or spinning is another. The point of these cross-training exercise opportunities is to take a break from the motion of running and the shock this activity creates for your legs. Keep in mind, though, that ellipticals and cycles utilize many of the same muscle groups, so they won't address the issue of muscle imbalance. These are also activities that involve no lateral (side to side) movement whatsoever. Consider other options as well, like plyometrics or high intensity interval training as a means of giving yourself a break from running. These can be great group activities to share with others. In our town, for instance, there's a gym (shout out to Jeremy and Heather over at Core Dynamix) that specializes in plyometrics and 'boot camp' training.

Give yourself a break from running and try some of these other options. You'll find the ones you like. Once you do, incorporate them regularly and you'll improve your chances of staying in top shape for running.

Body Strength Exercises

In addition to cross-training you should consider strengthening exercises on a regular basis. There are a number of easy body weight exercises you can do in the comfort of your own home that are based on compound movements that engage multiple muscle groups. What's more, these exercises engage OTHER muscle groups apart from the ones you use to run. The more well-developed muscle you have, the more you're able to burn fat efficiently. Remember, burning fat isn't about weight loss, but rather the idea of burning fuel in your body at a lower (and sustainable) rate of consumption over a period of time instead of tapping right into your body's glycogen stores. We store energy in our muscles, but only so much. But if we DO tap into the energy stored in our muscles, it stands to reason that having MORE muscle means having more energy to tap into.

There are a few exercises I'd recommend doing daily because they're going to be a great way of increasing your muscle mass through compound exercises. What are compound exercises? They're the ones that provide your body with an opportunity to utilize more than one muscle group to accomplish them. Here's a short list for you:

Plank
Push-ups
Sit-ups or crunches
Pull-ups (you'll need a bar for these)
Air squats

The exercises above are all body weight exercises. Even pull-ups, which technically require specialized equipment (a bar) do not require weights. You ARE the weight. If you do have weights and access to specialized machines, your options become endless. For now, though, I'd recommend keeping it simple and sticking to body weight exercises. There are a number of different websites and apps you can check out that include plans on how to increase your number of reps per day. Want to challenge yourself? Try a 100 push-ups challenge. You can do whatever you want here to keep things interesting, but the point is that you're engaging in an activity other than running ultimately for the sake of making your running easier and therefore more enjoyable!

Focusing on the Core

A strong core is especially important because it helps to give us a place to 'push' from. Though we're using our legs to run, we're essentially engaging in a controlled fall. We lean forward, we move around (if we're trying to navigate objects in our way) and we are using our diaphragm to breathe. Breathing becomes easier with a stronger core, and running is much more enjoyable when it feels easier. If you're not going to focus on anything else for strength training, at least focus on your core.

Stretching - Dynamic Versus Static

One final word on the idea of non-running movement - stretching. You'll see plenty of people engaging in pre-run stretching. Go to any 5K and watch people getting ready. There are two types of stretches you can engage in and one is very good before you run while one is very bad. VERY bad.

Static stretching - holding a muscle at a stretched point for a period of time and releasing.

Dynamic - stretching the muscle through repetitive motion.

Think about the difference between bending over and touching your toes and holding that position, or about sitting and doing a butterfly stretch. Which one is better? Or stated a different way - which one has the potential to injure you more than the other? Here's the answer – easy dynamic stretches BEFORE, and static stretches AFTER. Don't stretch and hold cold muscles. You run the risk of over-extending the muscles and of also damaging connective tissue. If you like static stretching more than dynamic, that's fine. Just warm up first. Go for a 5 to 10-minute easy run. Once you get your muscles warmed up, then engage in some static stretches.

Don't stretch and hold cold muscles. I'll say it one more time, for those out there who might benefit from repetition.

Chapter 8

Equipment and Hydration

There are no limits. There are only plateaus. But you must not stay there. You must go beyond them.

-Bruce Lee

Week 8 Overview

Pace	*Start Time*	*End Time*
Walk	0	2:00
Run	2:00	32:00:00
Intervals:	1	
Walk	1 minute	
Run	30 minutes	
Total run time	30 minutes	
Total walk time	2 minutes	

Footwear

Oh, the places we can go if we start talking about footwear. There are so many options out there, the choices to new runners are seemingly endless. What's worse, everyone and their mother (if their mother runs, and even sometimes if their mother *doesn't* run) is going to have their take on who makes the best shoes. Pros will endorse certain shoes. Other shoe manufacturers will tout their shoes as helping you accomplish specific running goals.

Want to know a secret? Lean in close, because I'm only telling *you*. You're in the inner circle and I want to make sure you have the key to figuring out which running shoe is the ideal running shoe for you. Are you ready?

It's all crap.

Do you know how much money shoe manufacturers pump into advertising? A lot. Do you know how much they pump into research and development? Also a lot. And do you know how much money shoe manufacturers (the big ones) *make* in a given year? More than enough to justify the amount they spend on marketing, offset by their R&D costs. Don't get me wrong. There are some great shoes out there. But the idea that what one person knows to be a great shoe will without fail work for another runner? That's the part that's crap. We all have our own unique biomechanics. While shoe A might work for Joe, shoe A might very well create a repetitive motion injury for Bob because Bob needs a stability shoe. Which shoe A most definitely is not.

Does the idea of different shoes based on different biomechanics have your head spinning yet? If not, start throwing in the idea of different midsole material depending on desired cushion density. Or different upper materials for different types of wear. And now, save yourself a lot of time and heartache and...

Go to a running store.

But wait, Nick. Are you saying that the pros are wrong? My friend is wrong? My *mother* is *wrong*? But she's never wrong. Just ask her!

Settle down. It might very well be the case that your friend's shoe recommendation works for you. But consider how much better it might be for you to go to a place where they can look at how you run and identify specific shoe recommendations that might work better for you. That sounds a lot better than a shot in the dark, right? They'll look at your gait (a fancy word for the way you run), look at how your feet are hitting the ground and whether you are neutral or overpronate or under-pronate, and some will even consider how hard your feet are hitting the ground and have recommendations for types of shoes based on cushioning and midsole/outsole construction.

Pretty cool, huh? Do yourself a favor and go talk to the knowledgeable folks at your local running store. You'll even run the risk of making a friend or two while you're there.

Barefoot Running

Born to Run (McDougall, 2011) was a book that came out a number of years ago and laid absolute waste to the idea of cushioned running shoes as being something we need. It ushered in the idea of a minimal shoe trend by stating that technology was actually working against us when it came to shoes. More cushioning was, instead of protecting our feet from damaging impact, having an opposite effect of allowing us to put even more impact pressure on our legs. Support from underneath was damaging our foot's ability to work as its own shock absorption system. The book focused on an ancient tribe of raramuri (the running people - the

Tarahumara) that ran just next to barefoot, using nothing more than pieces of rubber made into sandals to protect their feet from rocks.

And it is all true. Everything the book mentions is absolutely factual.

Here's the problem though. Two problems, actually, but both come to the same end. Let's break them down. First, from an early age most of us wear shoes. Our bodies develop while utilizing cushioning to 'protect' our legs and feet. Second, we have man-made surfaces to contend with. Running on concrete or asphalt is a very different thing from running on grass or dirt. These man-made surfaces, combined with the fact that we are accustomed to using our legs when we have cushioned shoes attached to our feet, mean we put ourselves at risk if we suddenly decide to adopt barefoot running.

That's not to say we can't be barefoot runners. Quite the opposite. I think when it comes down to it, we could ALL be barefoot runners. But we have to recondition our bodies a little at a time. And we also have to consider things like broken glass - a very quick way to ruin a great barefoot run. These are part of a larger category of things we'll call 'man-made obstacles' that will impede our ability to simply cast off our shoes and go for a run. But you can embrace your inner Tarahumara and still go barefoot. Companies like Xero shoes make minimal footwear that protect your feet but still allow you to engage in barefoot running motion. Give them a try. I've gone to extremes with my own minimal running, but I have come back to running shoes given time because of the additional protection they afford from the elements mainly.

Cushioning

So too much cushioning can be a bad thing, but then barefoot running can be something that anyone can do? How much more mixed messaging can you give?

You weren't listening. Or maybe I wasn't explaining it right. Let me try a different approach.

When you go to a running store, they're going to fit you into the shoe that works for you. Depending on your level of running experience (which is likely little to none if this will be your first time buying running shoes) you're going to want to listen to what they have to say about cushioning. Your body is not ready for barefoot running right out of the gate. If you aspire to run barefoot you can begin to ease yourself into that, but for now consider that cushioning is going to help to minimize some of the potential for impact damage. You're a new runner, and your form won't be great. You'll be hitting the ground harder with your feet. Running will tune you in to exactly how bad your form might be, or how hard you might be hitting the ground, and from there you'll improve. During all of this, your midsole cushioning will help to keep you safe. Cushioning isn't the evil thing it has been made out to be. One thing cushioning does have the capacity to do is to allow you to run with poor form without hurting yourself (or putting yourself at as much risk for injury). So use your cushioning but do so safely. Pay attention to how you run, and once you've been doing it for a while try to move down to more minimal cushioning and see how you do. You might find your form improves even more.

Stability

One other thing shoes can do is stabilize your foot if you turn your ankle in or out when you run. I'm talking about the bottom of your foot. If you engage in a regular range of motion with your foot you are referred to as 'neutral.' If your feet bend in when you run, it is called supination. If your feet bend out when you run, it is called pronation. Shoes can help to correct issues with supination and pronation by providing stability and motion control. Orthotics (inserts you put in your shoes) can be prescribed as well. If you're having ankle problems, foot problems, or pain you think might be caused by the way your feet are hitting the ground, get checked out. Stability can go a long way in making your runs more enjoyable and your running health more sustainable.

Just remember, as you're thinking about all of these things I've just thrown at you - you can't run if you're injured. The name of the game, when it comes to footwear, is to first and foremost work to prevent injury.

Hydration Packs

As with running shoes, there are lots of great products out there that you can begin to look at investing in as you increase your running distance and time. Hydration packs are specialized packs that either contain a bladder (a rubber bag with a tube you use to draw water from while you're running) or bottles, along with other things like energy gels, keys, phone, toilet paper (hopefully you won't ever need it, but better to be prepared), or anything else that might be something worth having for a longer distance run. There's a fine line between packing a few necessary items and packing for disaster preparedness on a TEOTWAWKI (the end of the world as we know it) scale. The lighter you pack, the less you'll be burdening yourself with heavy things you might not even use while you're on the run.

Which brings me to my point about hydration packs. Consider how long you're running, and whether you even need something like this. It can be handy to run with your keys or your phone, or maybe even a small water bottle, but you can easily overdo it. If you're only running for a few miles, or for under an hour total, I'd say leave the pack at home. Enjoy the run without having to carry around a bunch of extra weight. If you're fueling right during the day, you should be able to run for up to an hour without having to worry about refueling. Keep a water bottle available at your destination but approach the idea of packing and carrying with some reluctance, if possible.

Fads

When my wife and I were running triathlons regularly, one of the fads we continued to come across was elastic laces. These took on many forms, but the premise was basically the same. Instead of having to tie your shoes, you just converted them to slip-ons with the substitution of elastic lacing or bands. Great in theory, but I never ended up finding a setup that worked for me. In spite of trying a few different brands. I gave them a fair try, but they just weren't for me.

Some equipment fads will result in new products that will work wonders for you and will address a need you might not even be aware you had. Others will not pan out, and they'll result in you parting with more of your hard-earned money than you otherwise should have spent on such a silly product (always something you'll realize in hindsight, mind you, never when you are actually deciding to buy said products in the first place). Approach these 'fad' purchases carefully but do so with the realization that in some instances they might actually make your life better. I use the word fad to describe these products, but 'gimmick' is another word that comes to mind.

Road ID

For years now I have had a Road ID and I've worn it whenever I run. The idea is that when you run you should have some identification on you in case anything happens and you're incapacitated. People get hit by cars. It happens. People experience medical emergencies. If you're found on the side of the road, emergency responders need to know who you are and how they can reach your emergency contact(s). They also need to know if you have a pre-existing medical condition. Perhaps you're diabetic. Epileptic. Maybe you have a heart condition. These are the sorts of things that, if emergency responders know them, can greatly improve your chances of receiving the care you need when you need it. Consider getting some sort of identification you can carry with you that will help you when you most need it.

And not to end this chapter on a morbid note, but consider being an organ donor. We run because we like to run, and because it helps to keep us healthy. If anything *does* happen to you, there are so many out there who would benefit from the healthy organs you might be able to provide. Help a brother or sister out and pay it forward so that your running will be able to benefit others in an amazing way.

Chapter 9

What's Next?

Often when you think you're at the end of something, you're at the beginning of something else

-Fred Rogers

Setting Long-Term Goals

Now that you're running regularly, what is on your bucket list? Do you aspire to run your first 5K? Maybe you want to set your sights on something like a half-marathon or a marathon? These are all goals you can reach. The most important thing about goals is to decide on what they actually are, and then once you have them on paper you can begin to create a plan for how to get successfully from point A to point B.

Goals need to be realistic. If you want to run a marathon but you're just taking up running, I won't lie to you - it is going to be a while before you get there. Is it unreasonable? Of course not. But a marathon for a new runner is a goal that might involve a number of intermediate goals first, stepping stones along the way. 'Don't bite off more than you can chew' is an adage we've all heard before. Truth is, runners can 'chew' on an awful lot when it comes to establishing a base level of fitness. I have run half-marathon distances without any training beyond being able to run 3 miles regularly. Was it comfortable? Did I have fun? No, and also no. When you're considering your goals, you need to do so with the intent of making them fun to attain. You want to enjoy the time you're spending running that race you've planned for and trained for. You don't want to feel like every step is going to be your last. Put in the time and train right. There are TONS of training plans out there, for pretty much whatever distance you want to run. Yeah, even you, you crazy ultrarunners. Want to run a 100K? A 100 miler? Even those come with their own guidelines and recommendations.

Set your goals and dig deep. And if you don't want to run a marathon right now (or ever), that in no way makes you less of a runner than the next person who wants to run a marathon. You're running, and the key now is to keep yourself motivated. Running faster and running further are the two ways to move towards these goals you're going to be setting for yourself.

Increasing Speed

Increasing speed will be the first of your two goals. How do you do this? There are two ways. First, you'll want to keep track of your heart rate based on consistent running. If you continue to build your base level of fitness by abiding by your target heart rate, you'll continue to improve in speed. You'll be able to push yourself more and still stay below this target threshold. The other way you can increase speed is through interval training, which we'll talk about in a moment. The key here is consistency. You'll build fitness over time if you are running regularly based on the schedule you set for yourself. This is going to require that you put in more than a day or two a week. Increasing speed will come from base fitness that is built from running 3 to 5 times per week. CONSISTENTLY.

Increasing Distance

The formula you should use to calculate the amount of additional running you can add on in a week is generally agreed upon as 10%. That's a guideline, and it is also important to consider increases within the context of your skill level. Are you a beginning runner? You're not going to want to add on 10% every week. That's a recipe for injury, and you'll run the risk of sidelining yourself while you recover. Here's a simple breakdown:

Experienced runner - 10% increase every 1 to 2 weeks
Novice runner - 10% increase every 3 to 4 weeks

The best way to increase distance is to add this additional run volume proportionally to your tempo runs and your long run. We'll talk about types of running in the next session, with interval training, but let's look at a specific example. Say this is your training:

Monday - 3 miles
Wednesday - 3 miles
Saturday - 4 miles
Total miles - 10

In this example, there are runs on three different days and the Saturday run is the 'long' run. If you add an increase in run volume to this plan, you'd be adding 1 mile (because 3+3+4 = 10, and 10% of 10 is 1). You have options with how you can add this volume into your routine, but I'd recommend adding 0.25 to the Monday and Wednesday runs, and 0.5 to the Saturday run. The new schedule based on this increase would be:

Monday - 3.25
Wednesday - 3.25
Saturday - 4.5
Total miles - 11

The next increase, you might want to add the entire 10% to
your long run. It depends on your running goals. Also, if
you're adding distance during the week it means you're
adding time. You may not have the luxury of additional time
during the week, but you do on those weekend days when
you're doing a long run. Add the volume there, if you'd like.
The important thing is not to overdo increases in volume.
Give your body a chance to adjust and then listen to your
body if your heart rate is maxing out during the runs. This is
particularly true of your long runs. For long runs, follow the
rule of long slow distance (LSD). Your heart rate should be
lower because your pace should be lower.

Interval Training

Intervals are where things start to get fun. What is an
interval? A period of faster running followed by a period of
slower running (rest) that pushes you beyond your
regular/average running pace. Beyond that, it can be
anything. You can do intervals on a track, on a treadmill, or
on your regular run course. You're limited only by your
imagination. I'd recommend one interval session per week,
and generally not more than two. Here's a suggestion for an
interval session, based on a person whose average speed is 6
miles per hour (a 10-minute pace):

5 minute warmup run at 6 miles per hour
30 second sprint at 7 miles per hour

1 minute rest at 5 miles per hour
(repeat the 30 second sprint and the 1 minute rest 4 times)
5 minute cooldown at 5 miles per hour

That's the simplest approach. Decide on the number of intervals you want to start with, the speed you want to run them at, and give yourself a reasonable amount of rest between intervals. Warm up before you do them, and cool down afterwards. You're looking to push yourself. Ideally, you're looking for all-out effort on the sprints, but you can also improve your running speed through marginal gains. Just push yourself. And for building onto these interval sessions on a weekly basis you can add an additional sprint each week or try to increase your speed during the individual sprints.

Race Training and Tapering

If you're training for a specific distance in a race, you're going to follow a specific regimen. You're going to need to be consistent so you can peak at the right time. Your mileage and running volume will increase regularly over time if you're running a longer race, but your mileage may not reach the distance you'll be racing during any one run. In other words, if you're training for a marathon, you're generally not going to run a marathon distance until the race. You'll have long runs that get you close, but the idea with your training is that you'll be building strength over time and ability to run when you're already experiencing some form of fatigue. Many running plans for marathons will include back to back long runs, to simulate the difficulty you'll have in covering the distance during a race. The trick to training is that you're not putting yourself in a position where you're running such high volumes that you're having to take significant time off between your runs. You're reaching a high volume at the right time, and then you're tapering for the race. A taper occurs in your last few weeks leading up to the race. Your run volume will decrease, and you'll begin to take it easy so you can store up your energy for race day.

Periodization and Step Training

If you're not preparing for a specific race and you're simply running on a regular basis, I recommend practicing some form of periodization or step training. It will allow you to obtain gains in speed and distance over time safely and will provide your body with time to adjust to increases in volume.

Here's one scenario. You're increasing your distance every 2 weeks by 10%. Over the course of 8 weeks here are your running totals:

Week 1 and 2 - 10 miles
Weeks 3 and 4 - 11 miles
Weeks 5 and 6 - 12.1 miles
Weeks 7 and 8 - 13.3 miles

Now, you can continue to increase your running volume based on this regular 10% increase in a linear format, but periodization provides a different approach. It slows things down a little bit.

Weeks 1 and 2 - 10 miles
Weeks 3 and 4 - 11 miles
Weeks 5 and 6 - 12.1 miles
Weeks 7 and 8 - 11 miles

Weeks 9 and 10 - 12.1 miles
Weeks 11 and 12 - 13.3 miles
Weeks 13 and 14 - 12.1 miles
Weeks 15 and 16 - 13.3. Miles

I carried this volume increase out an additional 8 weeks to better illustrate the increases over time. You're adding distance in increments, and then backing off before moving forward. This provides your body with an opportunity to rest and to come back stronger. Up through week 6 we're increasing at our regular 10% rate. During weeks 7 and 8, instead of jumping up again by 10% we actually go back to the volume we ran in weeks 3 and 4. It is going to feel easy and there's a good reason why - we're giving our bodies a break.

Muscle is built during periods of rest. We engage in activities that stress our muscles and it is when they heal that they are built. Running is no different. If you just continue to increase and increase and increase without giving yourself a break, you're going to have a harder and harder time sustaining your effort. If you're increasing your run volume each week, do so according to some schedule of periodization. What I've outlined is only an example. You might opt to follow a different schedule, but I'd suggest increasing volume regularly for a period of time over 3 to 4 periods, and then backing off. You'll actually be able to make more progress over time and leapfrog forward much more effectively!

Sharing Your Accomplishments with Others

Be proud of your accomplishments. Share them if you'd like. There are plenty of other people out there who might benefit from your positive approach to running. We benefit as a community from hearing about others' successes and failures. We learn as a group based on our collective experiences. Sharing your accomplishments is a great way of putting your experiences out there for others to learn. It is also a great way of keeping track of your own victories and using them as a measurement as you continue to work to improve your running.

You don't have to keep this information in a public format. You can keep these remarks to yourself, but I would recommend that you write them down. If you don't end up sharing them, at least you can have them as a reference for yourself. If you had a good race or a bad race, if you had a good training session or ended up injuring yourself, it is helpful to be able to go back to what you were doing at that time to try to figure out what happened to produce those results. If you're sharing this information with a larger audience, they might even be able to provide input on what happened and see something in your training or racing that you missed.

Being an Extrovert

Some people like to advertise their running by wearing it on their sleeve, literally. They'll want to wear race shirts all the time, they'll want to talk to other people about running, they'll keep their longest race distances plastered on their cars, and they'll be... a bit too much for the non-runners to handle sometimes. Running is funny like that. You'll find, perhaps, that over time you are more and more culturally ingrained in running, and it is something that is part of who 'you' are. I go back and forth. I'm very extroverted sometimes when I talk to others about running and present myself as a runner. I'm also very solitary about my own approach and downplay how much I actually love running because I don't want to be overwhelming to people who don't feel the same way. You'll figure out how you feel about it over time, and how much you want to let people out there know you're a runner. Keep in mind though, that your enthusiasm for talking about running or showing people what you've been able to accomplish might motivate others to run. And what a great thing that would be. Friends, family, even people you don't know - they might draw inspiration from you and want to begin their own journey to running.

Chapter 10

Running Stories

Have you ever run with a drunk man before?

Random drunk man running at midnight in downtown Chicago

Chicago and Running at Loyola

I was deep into a run streak when I had a business trip in Chicago. Running at that time was non-negotiable. I ran every day, and that was that. In order to do that, I ended up needing to be creative about how I scheduled the runs. Friday night I ran, and I knew I'd be busy on Saturday, so I stayed up until after midnight on Friday, AFTER having run 8 miles. I went out and did another two miles and had one of the most memorable encounters I've ever had on a run, with a random drunk guy. In downtown Chicago. At about 1 in the morning.

(Journal entry from Friday, June 2, 2017 - day 521 of run streak)

When you run, you see things other people just don't have an opportunity to see. You drive by in a car, with the windows rolled up, and you're oblivious to what is going on in the world around you. You ride a bike and it gets a little better, but you're still whizzing by too fast to see things sometimes. You run, and the only thing you have are your two feet and the speed they take you along at. You're an active participant in the environment around you. You're not just a passive observer. You dodge dogs, run through traffic, jump over obstacles and experience whatever Mother Nature throws at you.

Tonight was one of those nights. In all my years of running I've only had a few runs that I'd consider to be particularly memorable. Just as there are runs I'll never remember again (miles 16 through 24 of my first marathon, for example) there are runs I'll never forget. Running during sunrise in San Diego - 9 miles. Running my first Big Lake Half - in around 1:51. The first 20 miles of Vermont 50 (I dropped at mile 35 - it stands as my only DNF in a race... ever). And perhaps my favorite memorable run of them all, a late-night run with Merrie after a few hours of substantial drinking with our friends Eric and Stephanie.

Good running moments don't come along often. Tonight was one though. I didn't get up and run early, so I knew I'd have my work cut out for me tonight. I am on a business trip in Chicago and it wasn't until around 9pm that I got back to my room after dinner. I called home and talked to Merrie and Jack, and I texted Alex. I was out the door by about 9:30, and I went 1 mile down on Sheridan to the Lake Front trail. Did 3 more miles out on the trail, then 4 miles back to the room for a total of 8 in a fairly brisk 1:12. On Sheridan I passed a park where everyone was sitting in lawn chairs, watching Young Frankenstein. When I turned onto the bike path there was a guy over in a clearing juggling neon LED-lit bowling pins. Red, green orange, blue, just swirling around seemingly by themselves. Further down the path I heard giggling and saw a playground on my left, filled with kids running around playing in the dark. Lincoln Park down the path, and lit tennis courts. Perfect weather. No wind. Just a magical run. I have a special place in my heart for runs like those.

"Have you ever run with a drunk man before?"

There was actually only about an hour between yesterday's run and today's run. I got in two more miles shortly after midnight so I wouldn't break my running streak. My knees were really feeling it, so I cut short what I had originally estimated might become another 4 to 6 miles. I did a mile out on Sheridan, turned around, and then headed back on the opposite side of the road. Ahead of me about 200 feet was a guy, just kind of walking along. As I passed him on the left, he broke into a stumbling jog and kept pace with me. I wasn't going very fast. About 10:30. I had pepper spray on me, and we were in a very well-lit and heavily populated area, and I knew there were three police officers about a quarter mile ahead of me. Someone had run off the road and knocked over a light pole, so they were taping off the area. The guy didn't say anything for a little while, then he turned to me and said, "Have you ever run with a drunk man before?" Jamaican guy (judging from his heavy accent), skinny, fairly well dressed, just running along with me keeping my pace. I said I couldn't remember whether I'd ever run with any drunk people before, but I'd run before when I was drunk myself. He chatted back and forth with me, asking me why I ran. I tried to explain it to him, but he just wasn't getting it. I tried to explain the fact that I run every day, and not running for one day is just not an option. That I was running at midnight so I could be sure I was getting my miles in for the day. He kept pace, kept chatting, and then when we reached Loyola I turned, and he continued running on his merry way.

Make that two memorable runs in two days. Can't say I remember that ever happening before.

San Diego

I decided to start a run streak at the end of 2015, and once I made a deliberate decision to run every day, I started to reap the rewards by gaining speed and distance. I went to San Diego in March of 2016 for another business trip, and this was a particularly memorable run. I was staying at a Hilton right on the bay, and there was a waterfront path that was well-maintained. I had run on it the previous day and decided on a whim to get up and do a long run while I was there.

(Journal entry from Friday, March 25, 2016 - day 85 of run streak)

Duele mucho. I just did 9 around the bay. I had intended to be up by 5 but I slept in until 5:30. I got up and choked down half of a protein bar and I was on my way. Around mile 4 I hit a bit of a wall, and another one around mile 6. The last two miles hurt but they went fairly quickly. A few issues on the run, but nothing major. I didn't wear a tight enough undershirt, so my nipples are chafed up. Fueling was good. I had a GU at 4.5 miles, and that kept me going.

Watching the sun come up is always an enjoyable thing when running. I thought seeing the sun rise over San Diego was pretty cool. It was one of those runs that will be memorable. Not epic, just memorable. San Diego is just so quiet compared to other cities. If I had to pick a word to describe the morning, it was surreal.

Running Around DC

This was a tough one to capture in words. I was at the end of my rope finishing my dissertation and was beyond stressed with pretty much everything in my life. It was a much-needed run just for being able to get out and focus on other things for a little while, and to try to forget everything I had going on. It is a good one to read again because it reminds me that running, if you make it a priority, can be a good thing. And it should be a priority. For me, it was something that truly helped me through.

I had just pulled an all-nighter while I was on a trip in DC, and decided I needed to just get a good run into my system to flush out all the stress.

(Journal entry from Friday, September 30, 2016 - day 275 of run streak)

Things will get better, I keep telling myself. There is light at the end of the tunnel. The best is right around the corner. All that crap we tell ourselves to remain positive. I was up until 5am last night / this morning trying to finish up another revision for another chapter of my dissertation. I'm nearly done in. I just need to be done.

I went for a run this morning down at the National Mall. It was the first time I really had any decent time to myself. I slept in until about 9:30 and I was on the road by about 10. It was a fairly crappy day weather-wise, but I have plenty of gear so that's not an issue. I took my Camelbak and I also had a credit card and some cash. I ended up grabbing lunch on the way home, instead of my original plan of getting lunch at the sculpture garden over at the Mall. All good. I got kind of choked up on the run at a few points. Life just gets to be a little too much to process sometimes. I have a hard time dealing with things. I do the best I can, and that's the best I can do. I'll just try to keep moving forward and work on getting through the tough times.

Tomorrow I fly back to NH. I'm dreading getting the email from my dissertation chair on additional edits, but I think being so close to the defense date they have no choice other than to allow me to defend. I'm going to try to work on it for a little while tomorrow before I get on the plane. I've got plenty of time, and if I just plan to leave here early and head to the airport then there won't be any potential distractions. I'll take tomorrow night off to spend with the family, then it looks like another marathon writing session on Sunday. This time it will be my dissertation defense presentation.

Other than that, life just moves forward. I did another run tonight so I could see what the monuments looked like at night. It was crappy weather, but I Facetimed with Jack and Alex while I was at the National Mall. That was kind of neat. I'm going to maybe pack one or two more things tonight and then just call it, I think. I'm done.

Other Stories

I'm an avid journal keeper, but sometimes there are stories I neglect to write down. For instance, there was one memorable New Year's Eve that we decided it would be a good idea to go for a run right before midnight. As I recall, we were on a running streak and had to get in our miles before the day was over, but we had gone over to see our friends Eric and Stephanie. As it was New Year's Eve, I had a few drinks and was in a particularly celebratory mood by the time we went for a run. Around 11:30. It was pitch black out, but Merrie and I had flashlights, so we went out and logged a quick out-and-back run of about a mile and a half total. I was 'enthusiastic' about the run, and by Merrie's account I was being loud and obnoxious, declaring it to be the 'best run ever' and going on and on about how much I love running in the dark. And about how we should do this sort of thing more often.

For the record, I generally *don't* like running in the dark.

I've been hit by a car twice, but I can't find a record of that in any of my prior journal entries either. The first time was at the elementary school in town. It was the end of the school day and parents were picking their kids up. There's a very specific flow of traffic that occurs at the beginning and end of the day, with the two main driveways becoming one-way. One way in, and one way out. I was doing fine crossing the 'in' driveway but crossing the 'out' apparently the car didn't see me running across the driveway. She started to pull out and ran right into me. I wasn't hurt, but it was enough to get my attention. I stopped, turned and raised my hands to her and gave her one of those *"I'm walkin' here!"* looks. It could have been worse.

The second time I was running on our road and a car was coming at me. I was on the edge of the road because the section I was running had no shoulder. There are spots on our road whether vegetation overgrowth simply prevents you from being able to move over. With that said, cars should move over for runners. This is a thing that many drivers don't seem to understand. Instead there seems to be a *how dare you run on MY road* mentality. So I was running on the edge of the road, observing that the car wasn't moving over and trying to decide what to do. As the car came by, the passenger side window nailed me at about shoulder level. Which didn't feel very good since the car was doing about 40. Thankfully it was a glancing blow, but it was enough to get my attention!

That's the great thing about running. Not the fact that sometimes we get hit by cars, but that we have stories to tell. With the good runs and the bad runs, there are opportunities to make memories. We do the best we can in terms of running safely and in not putting ourselves at risk by doing stupid things like running without lights or reflective gear, but in spite of our best efforts some of our 'stories' might center around issues of injury as a result of our safety having been compromised. But we learn from these things. We run safer. We become more aware of our surroundings. We realize that what we do has some inherent risk, but that it is also an amazing activity that allows us to see those things we might otherwise miss.

References and Resources

One way you can invest time in improving your running, apart from actually spending time running, is to read. I've broken the books below into sections depending on focus, but there is some cross-pollination here. For example, in Scott Jurek's book "Eat and Run" he's been kind enough to include some great recipes. In "The 4 Hour Body" Tim Ferriss goes well beyond discussing diet and also give you great information on... pretty much anything else that impacts your health. Even in the fiction section, you can glean ideas for intervals and training plans from Denton and Cassidy. These books are only the tip of the iceberg, but without them you would not have the book you now hold in your hands. Each of these books has been instrumental to me one way or another, and in many instances I've referred to them directly in this book. I encourage you to consume them voraciously. I've also taken the liberty of including my own commentary on why these are such great books to read.

Food

Esselstyn, Rip (2017). **The Engine 2 Diet: The Texas Firefighter's 28-Day Save-Your-Life Plan that Lowers Cholesterol and Burns Away the Pounds.** Grand Central Life & Style.

Rip's book is an excellent read, in terms of outlining the benefits of a plant-based diet. It is also eye-opening in revealing the potential damage we're inflicting on ourselves by creating meat and dairy. Rip takes a very effective approach of including a number of testimonials from people who have tried his diet (which is not a diet but a lifestyle) and been successful. The lifestyle isn't for everyone, but it is definitely worth a try.

Ferriss, Timothy (2010). **The 4 Hour Body: An Uncommon Guide to Rapid Fat Loss, Incredible Sex and Becoming Superhuman.** Harmony.

To me, this book was life changing. Not because I had success through practicing what Tim has written about (although I did) but because of his approach. He breaks things down in such a way that he's looking for maximum return from minimal effort. This is a great all-around book for giving you a great path to follow regardless of how you're trying to improve yourself. I'd call this one an overall self-help book, but I think the chapters on food are particularly important. Hence my including it in the food section.

Harper, Bob (2012). **The Skinny Rules: The Simple, Nonnegotiable Principles for Getting to Thin.** Ballantine.

The title says it all. Nonnegotiable. If you want something, or if you have a goal you want to achieve, you need to be able to think in terms of non-negotiables. Bob establishes a very easy to follow set of rules that provide a great roadmap for making changes in your daily routines that will pay you dividends down the road by focusing your fueling habits on more effective consumption of food. Too often we tend to eat now and then feel bad about it later. Bob doesn't care if you feel bad. If you feel bad afterwards but keep screwing up and making bad choices, too bad for you. Bob is all about tough love and it really comes through in the way he's written this book.

Stone, Gene (2011). **Forks Over Knives: The Plant-Based Way to Health.** The Experiment.

Stone's book, like the Esselstyn book, touts the benefits of a plant-based diet. It is a good one to read if you're considering ways you might approach your eating with more awareness of what you're putting in your body and how it might be affecting you. I should say, after citing both of these books, that I am NOT a vegetarian as of the current writing of this book. I will say that these books have given me pause to consider if there are more effective ways I can and should be fueling my body.

Running Books from the Pros

Jurek, Scott (2012). **Eat & Run: My Unlikely Journey to Ultramarathon Greatness.** Houghton Mifflin Harcourt.

The Jerker is one of my heroes. Truly. This book is a great read and Scott has a wonderful sense of humor that shows through and really captures what it is like to experience the slog of ultramarathons. Even us mortal runners who only complete meager distances can learn a lot by his credo: Sometimes you just do things.

Karnazes, Dean (2005). **Ultramarathon Man: Confessions of an All-Night Runner.** Tarcher Perigree.

Karno is a crazy guy, and many would say that much of his motivation with presenting himself as an all-night runner has been for the sake of publicity and self-promotion. But isn't that sort of the point of writing an autobiographical book? To publicize and self-promote yourself by telling everyone your story? Regardless, it makes for an amusing read as Dean spins his tale about how he came to running later in life and just kept running. And running.

Hall, Ryan (2011). **Running with Joy: My Daily Journey to the Marathon.** Harvest House Publishers.

Ryan literally breaks it down into individual training days and sessions. Great stuff for illustrating exactly how much preparation goes into marathon training. I'm not a religious person so some of his discussion of spirituality is a bit lost on me, but he's an amazing marathoner and world-class athlete. And he's an all-around great guy.

Keflezighi, Meb (2015). **Meb for Mortals: How to Run, Think, and Eat Like a Champion Marathoner.** Rodale Books.

Meb is... Meb. Enough said. Read this book. Another unique set of insights into marathon training, sure, but this book also does a great job of capturing how life-encompassing training for a race can be. It isn't just the running you do. It is everything. It is the way you live your life.

Strength Training and Running Science

Maffetone, Philip (2010). **The Big Book of Endurance Training and Racing.** Skyhorse.

Those of us who run owe a debt of gratitude to Philip for his tireless efforts to document effective practices around training and racing. This is truly an amazing reference, and one I've gone to again and again.

McDougall, Christopher (2011). **Born to Run: A Hidden Tribe, Superathletes, and the Greatest Race the World has Never Seen.** Vintage.

This is the book that started it all, many say, when it comes to the idea of barefoot running. The book is a very motivating read, and it also introduced me to Scott Jurek for the first time. Entertaining, and it doesn't come across as preachy.

Fiction

Parker, Jr., John L. (1978). **Once a Runner.** Cedarwinds.

The first in a series of three books written by Parker chronicling the adventures of Quenton Cassidy. Quenton is a Prefontaine-esque character whose training is largely overseen by Bruce Denton (a Frank Shorter-esque character in his own right). Chronologically this is the middle of the story, but I recommend reading them in order of release.

Parker, Jr., John L. (2008). **Again to Carthage.** Breakaway Books.

Again to Carthage picks up where Once a Runner left off.

Parker, Jr., John L. (2015). **Racing the Rain: A Novel.** Scribner.

Racing the Rain takes the story back to Cass's beginnings as a junior high and high school runner in Florida.

Appendices

Chart for Distances and Times

If you're interested in calculating how far you're actually running based on your speed and overall time, here is a chart for you that gives you distance based on interval. When does this come in handy? Say you're running for 17 minutes at 5 miles per hour. How far is that? How about wanting to know how fast you have to run in order to run a mile in 12 minutes? The chart can be revealing if you're looking at how increases in speed can impact your distance over time!   The speeds I've used here span from 1 mile per hour to 8 miles per hour, and from 1 minute of run time to 30. If what you're doing falls outside of these parameters (if you're running over 30 minutes or faster than 8 miles per hour) there are some great online calculators you'll be able to find fairly easily - just search "distance speed time" and you'll find calculators that let you solve for one of these numbers when you have the other two.

Time	1 mph	2 mph	3 mph	4 mph
1 minute	0.016	0.033	0.05	0.067
1 minute 30 seconds	0.025	0.05	0.075	0.1
2 minutes	0.033	0.066	0.1	0.133
3 minutes	0.05	0.1	0.15	0.2
4 minutes	0.066	0.133	0.2	0.267
5 minutes	0.083	0.166	0.25	0.333
6 minutes	0.1	0.2	0.3	0.4
7 minutes	0.116	0.233	0.35	0.467

8 minutes	0.133	0.266	0.4	0.533
9 minutes	0.15	0.3	0.45	0.6
10 minutes	0.167	0.333	0.5	0.667
11 minutes	0.183	0.366	0.55	0.733
12 minutes	0.2	0.4	0.6	0.8
13 minutes	0.216	0.433	0.65	0.867
14 minutes	0.233	0.466	0.7	0.933
15 minutes	0.25	0.5	0.75	1
16 minutes	0.267	0.533	0.8	1.067
17 minutes	0.283	0.566	0.85	1.133
18 minutes	0.3	0.6	0.9	1.2
19 minutes	0.316	0.633	0.95	1.267
20 minutes	0.333	0.666	1	1.333
21 minutes	0.35	0.7	1.05	1.4
22 minutes	0.367	0.733	1.1	1.467
23 minutes	0.383	0.766	1.15	1.533
24 minutes	0.4	0.8	1.2	1.6
25 minutes	0.416	0.833	1.25	1.667
26 minutes	0.433	0.866	1.3	1.733
27 minutes	0.45	0.9	1.35	1.8
28 minutes	0.466	0.933	1.4	1.867
29 minutes	0.483	0.966	1.45	1.933
30 minutes	0.5	1	1.5	2

Time	5 mph	6 mph	7 mph	8 mph
1 minute	0.083	0.1	0.117	0.133
1 minute 30 seconds	0.125	0.15	0.175	0.2
2 minutes	0.167	0.2	0.233	0.267
3 minutes	0.25	0.3	0.35	0.4
4 minutes	0.333	0.4	0.466	0.533
5 minutes	0.416	0.5	0.583	0.666
6 minutes	0.5	0.6	0.7	0.8
7 minutes	0.583	0.7	0.816	0.933
8 minutes	0.667	0.8	0.933	1.066
9 minutes	0.75	0.9	1.05	1.2
10 minutes	0.833	1	1.167	1.333
11 minutes	0.916	1.1	1.283	1.466
12 minutes	1	1.2	1.4	1.6
13 minutes	1.083	1.3	1.516	1.733
14 minutes	1.167	1.4	1.633	1.867
15 minutes	1.25	1.5	1.75	2
16 minutes	1.333	1.6	1.866	2.133
17 minutes	1.416	1.7	1.983	2.266
18 minutes	1.5	1.8	2.1	2.4
19 minutes	1.583	1.9	2.216	2.533
20 minutes	1.667	2	2.333	2.667
21 minutes	1.75	2.1	2.45	2.8
22 minutes	1.833	2.2	2.566	2.933
23 minutes	1.916	2.3	2.683	3.066
24 minutes	2	2.4	2.8	3.2

25 minutes	2.083	2.5	2.916	3.333
26 minutes	2.167	2.6	3.033	3.466
27 minutes	2.25	2.7	3.15	3.6
28 minutes	2.333	2.8	3.266	3.733
29 minutes	2.416	2.9	3.383	3.866
30 minutes	2.5	3	3.5	4

Chart of Speed Combinations

Here are some suggested training plans you can utilize depending on what speed you're running at and what speed you're walking at. I've titled them as introductory, intermediate, and advanced. One of the simplest ways to figure out what speed you should potentially run at while you're on the plan is to walk for 30 minutes and see how far you're walking in overall distance. Then refer to the chart above to get your speed in miles per hour. Once you have that, I would suggest generally adding about 2 miles per hour for your runs. This is easiest accomplished on a treadmill where you can program the equipment to run at a specific speed for a specific period of time, but it also works outside.

	Introductory	**Intermediate**	**Advanced**
	Walk at 2.5, run at 4	Walk at 3, run at 5	Walk at 4, run at 6
Week 1, distance per session	1.449	1.767	2.267
Week 2, distance per session	1.6	1.967	2.467
Week 3, distance per session	1.625	2	2.5
Week 4, distance per session	1.749	2.167	2.667
Week 5, distance per session	1.933	2.4	2.933

Week 6, distance per session	1.85	2.3	2.8
Week 7, distance per session	2.125	2.65	3.2
Week 8, distance per session	2.083	2.6	3.133

Target Heart Rate Zones

The chart below provides guidelines for max heart rate and target heart rate based on your age. The equation for calculating these heart rates is included in Chapter 5. To keep things simple, I've rounded the heart rates up or down in the target heart rate column to provide whole numbers as a guideline.

Age	Max Heart Rate	Target Heart Rate
16	204	163
17	203	162
18	202	162
19	201	161
20	200	160
21	199	159
22	198	159
23	197	158
24	196	157
25	195	156
26	194	155
27	193	154
28	192	154
29	191	153
30	190	152
31	189	151
32	188	150
33	187	150
34	186	149
35	185	148
36	184	147
37	183	146
38	182	146
39	181	145
40	180	144
41	179	143
42	178	142

43	177	142
44	176	141
45	175	140
46	174	139
47	173	138
48	172	138
49	171	137
50	170	136
51	169	135
52	168	134
53	167	134
54	166	133
55	165	132
56	164	131
57	163	130
58	162	130
59	161	129
60	160	128
61	159	127
62	158	126
63	157	126
64	156	125
65	155	124
66	154	123
67	153	122
68	152	122
69	151	121
70	150	120
71	149	119
72	148	118
73	147	118
74	146	117
75	145	116
76	144	115
77	143	114
78	142	114
79	141	113
80	140	112

Strength Training Chart - Suggested Exercises and Schedule

Here's a suggested schedule for incorporating strength training exercises into your regular regimen. This is based on body weight exercises and approaching a training plan based on three times per week strength training. You'll want to give yourself time off between training sessions, to let your muscles recover and develop. Remember, muscles develop during periods of rest! This plan also includes the types of runs (again... suggested runs) you'll be doing during the week.

	Running	**Strength Training**
Monday	Off	Off
Tuesday	Tempo Run	Arms and Core
Wednesday	Easy Run	Off
Thursday	Interval Run	Legs and Core
Friday	Cross training	Off
Saturday	Long Run	Off
Sunday	Easy Run	Core

Keep it even simpler if you'd like and create a circuit that incorporates muscle groups across your entire body, and then do the same circuit every day you do your strength training. It might look like this:

Pull-ups	3 sets of 10
Push-ups	3 sets of 10
Crunches	3 sets of 10
Plank	2 minutes
Air squats	3 sets of 10

You'll increase your reps over time, and you can accomplish your gains in a more linear way without having to worry about periodization because you're going to reach a threshold of overall reps. You can decide what your threshold might be. As with your running plan though, consistency is what you're shooting for. Here's a suggested increase schedule:

Week 1 - 3 sets of 10
Week 2 - 3 sets of 11
Week 3 - 3 sets of 12
Week 4 - 4 sets of 6
Week 5 - 4 sets of 7
Week 6 - 4 sets of 8
Week 7 - 4 sets of 9
Week 8 - 4 sets of 10
Week 9 - 4 sets of 11
Week 10 - 4 sets of 12
Week 11 - 5 sets of 6
Week 12 - 5 sets of 7
Week 13 - 5 sets of 8
Week 14 - 5 sets of 9
Week 15 - 5 sets of 10

In this example we see a starting point of 30 reps total in week 1, and an increase to 50 reps in week 15. You might increase in different ways, but the point of this example is to show that incremental gains can result in significant increases over time in overall repetitions.

ABOUT THE AUTHOR

Nick Marks lives in New England with his wife Merrie and his two sons, Alex and Jack, and a modest collection of four-legged animals including, at last count, two dogs and four cats. He enjoys writing both fiction and non-fiction. In his spare time, he promises to get around to house projects but never seems to be able to make any headway. Alas, his writing is proof of concept. So many ideas, and so little time. He can usually be found running around on the roads around his house, participating in various area races, coaching track, and running with the New Durham running group.